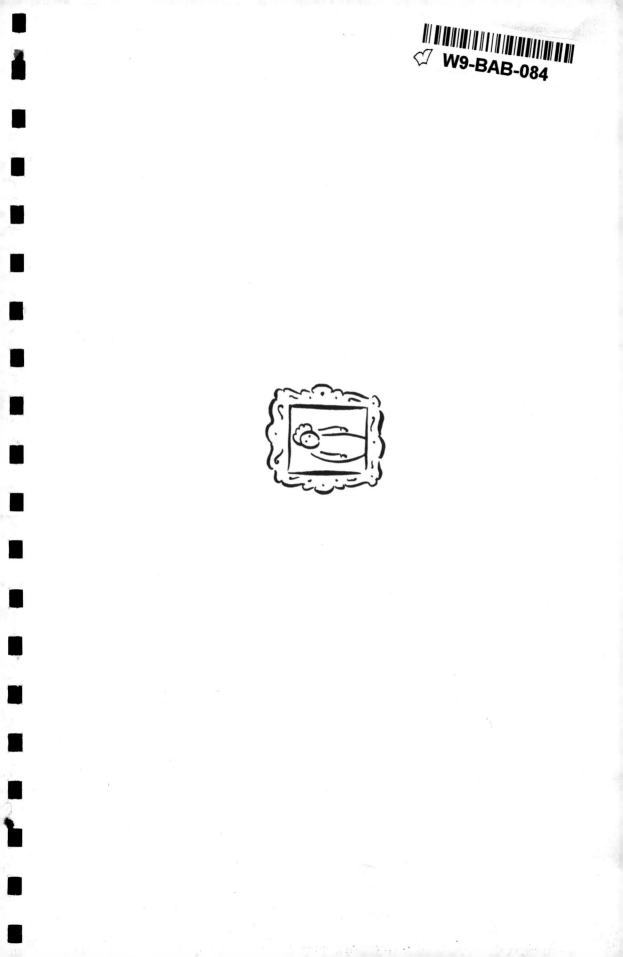

The Pregnancy Journal

*A Day-to-Day Guide
to a Healthy and Happy Pregnancy*

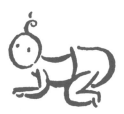

A. CHRISTINE HARRIS, PH.D.

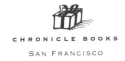

CHRONICLE BOOKS

SAN FRANCISCO

To my own precious family:
my husband, Bob, and my daughters, Heather and Wendy

Printed in Hong Kong.
Library of Congress Cataloging-in-Publication Data.

Harris, A. Christine
    The pregnancy journal : a day-to-day guide to a healthy and happy pregnancy
/ A. Christine Harris.
    p. cm.
    Includes index.
    ISBN 0-8118-1156-5
    1. Pregnancy—Popular works.   2. Pregnancy—Miscellanea.
    I. Title.
    RG525.H357   1996
    618.2'4—dc20   95-12870
                                    CIP

Book and cover design: Gretchen Scoble
Cover and interior illustration: Greg Stadler

Distributed in Canada by Raincoast Books
8680 Cambie Street
Vancouver, B.C. V6P 6M9

20 19 18 17 16 15 14 13 12 11

Chronicle Books
85 Second Street
San Francisco, CA 94105
www.chroniclebooks.com

CONTENTS

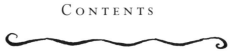

PREFACE

When I was pregnant with my two daughters, Heather (the eldest by three years) and Wendy, I was amazed by the transforming properties of pregnancy. I felt different, in many ways physically better than usual and "special" because I was carrying a child. But there were also some surprises: I felt unusually tired, even with normal rest, and I worried more than I thought I would. I was also surprised that I could apply so little of my knowledge about prenatal development and human behavior to my own pregnancy.

My practitioners offered good care, but their answers to my questions about my baby's development always seemed vague: "How's my baby doing?" I would ask. "Fine," they would say, "I can hear the baby's heartbeat." I longed to know more: What features were present? Could my baby move around? Was my baby processing any sensory information? How much did the baby weigh? Where was my baby in terms of development?

I eventually found the answers to these questions while doing research for a textbook on child development. Those answers, too late to provide insight into the chronology of my own pregnancies, are summarized within the pages of this book. Thus, it is my hope that *The Pregnancy Journal* will help parents-to-be feel knowledgeable, aware, and comfortable about the progress of their pregnancy and the development of their baby before birth. The journal can also become a keepsake to share with your baby when it's older and to help you compare your other pregnancies.

ACKNOWLEDGMENTS

Like pregnancy, writing a book is a labor of love, dedication, and hard work. I am grateful for the support, encouragement, and good advice of a fine collection of people: My sister, Carolyn Johnson, of Metro Design Center in San Jose, California, whose sample layout transformed lifeless text into an eye-catching document; my colleague Catherine Hooper, for her well-timed pregnancy, her personal warmth, and her "connections"; Rob Shaeffer and Karen Silver of Chronicle Books, for their interest in the project and their excellent editorial advice; Clyde Perlee, Jr., editor-in-chief of West Publishing Company, for his unfailing help and encouragement throughout the long incubation of this project; John Davis, for his many excellent ideas and his enthusiasm; Social Science/Humanities dean Bill Karns, for his consideration and good humor; good friends Karen Andrew, Cathy Kennedy, Barbara Mitchell, Becky Noon Schwarzer, and Cosumnes River College friends and colleagues for their strength; and Bob, Heather, and Wendy, for their patience and understanding.

Personalizing the Pregnancy Journal

All of the information in this journal is keyed to your specific due date. In that way, the information is not just a description of the sequence of events for any pregnancy, it's the sequence of events for your unique pregnancy.

The easiest way to personalize *The Pregnancy Journal* is to begin with your baby's estimated due date, Day 266. First, open the book to Day 266 (page 158) and write your baby's estimated due date on that day. Then, using a monthly calendar as a guide and working backward from Day 266, date each day in reverse sequence.

For example, if your baby is due on January 2:

Day 266 = January 2

Day 265 = January 1

Day 264 = December 31

Mark the days all the way back to Journal Day 1, the approximate day your baby was conceived.

For simplicity's sake, the medical profession actually counts the two weeks that set the stage for conception as part of "the pregnancy" by asking you to remember back to the first day of your last menstrual cycle. Thus, your doctor's estimate seems ahead by two weeks because of its earlier starting point. Going back 38 weeks from the baby's due date (266 days) takes you back to the estimated day of conception; going back 40 weeks from the baby's due date (280 days) takes you back to the first day of the woman's last menstrual cycle. In both cases, the due date remains the same.

Now that you have personalized your journal, you will be able to follow the unfolding events of your baby's development and your pregnancy by using the journal like a daily planner. You can read about your baby's growth for today's date, look ahead to see what you can expect, and look back to see what has already taken place.

Development is measured in Lunar Months.
Each month consists of 28 days organized into
four weeks of seven days each.

Lunar Month 1

THINGS TO DO THIS MONTH:

Eat a well-balanced diet of small, frequent meals and drink plenty of liquid.

Make sure you get 74-78 grams of protein a day and plenty of calcium.

Avoid foods that cause indigestion, heartburn, bloating, or other discomfort.

Don't drink alcohol (even beer and wine).

Get plenty of rest.

Exercise moderately.

Urinate when you feel the need.

Control nausea and stomach upset with natural, nondrug remedies.

Select a practitioner and contact them if you experience vaginal bleeding,
menstrual-like cramps, or lower abdominal pain.

week 1

DAY 1	DATE:
	265 days to go

Today, a single cell organism was formed from the union of your ovum, or egg, and your partner's sperm. Over the coming months, your daughter or son will develop from this barely visible single-cell, called a zygote. This beginning is called conception or fertilization.

As you think back, do you remember this date? Some women can feel when they ovulate, others can't. (It's okay either way.) It actually takes the sperm several hours to reach the egg. The egg is still usually within the Fallopian tube (the tube that connects the ovaries with the uterus) when the sperm begin to arrive. Although hundreds of sperm may swarm the egg, only one will penetrate the egg's outer surface. While this process of fertilization involves a tremendous amount of activity by the involved cells, you are as unaware of the event of fertilization as you are the routine production of red blood cells by your system or any other cellular event.

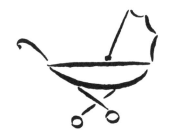

DAY 2	DATE:
	264 days to go

The first cell division takes place today. A two-sided ball is formed from the single cell created by your ovum and your partner's sperm.

Early Pregnancy Factor (EPF), an immuno-suppressant protein, is first manufactured now. Without EPF, your body might mistake the developing baby for a foreign body (like a bacterium or a virus) and attack it. With EPF, your baby can continue to develop without risk.

Chart your waist size and weight here. This first measurement is very important. You'll have fun looking back and comparing each of the measurements with the ones that preceded.

WAIST SIZE   WEIGHT

notes

....

....

....

....

....

....

....

....

....

....

Nothing is worth more than this day.

J. W. GOETHE

DAY 3	DATE: *263 days to go*

In the last twenty-four hours, the two identical cells have undergone three to four additional cell divisions. Two cells become four, four cells become eight, and eight cells become sixteen in a tightly packed, solid-ball configuration. Because the original cell is dividing into smaller units, there is little if any corresponding increase in your baby's total size.

The baby's cells are manufactured now by relying on the nutrients stored in the ovum that you produced.

DAY 4	DATE: *262 days to go*

The sixteen-cell solid ball has reached the end of your Fallopian tube and now enters your uterus.

The ball of cells that was once the egg is still too small to be seen. It has been floating freely on the fluids within your reproductive system.

notes

....

....

....

....

....

....

....

....

....

....

DAY 5	DATE: *261 days to go*

An important change takes place in the cell ball. Fluid passes into the center of the cell ball. The fluid divides the cells into two groups: those on the outside (these cells will form the placenta) and those on the inside (these cells will form the baby). The placenta is the organ that develops in the uterus at the site of implantation. Your blood circulates through the placenta and passes oxygen and nutrients to the baby while collecting blood-borne waste.

If the cell ball hasn't already entered your uterus, it will do so today. Your body still doesn't realize the baby exists, since EPF is secreted by the cell ball.

There is no finer investment for any community than putting milk into babies.
WINSTON CHURCHILL

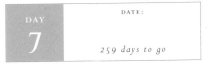

DAY **6**	DATE:
	260 days to go

If fluid hasn't already passed into the center of the cell ball to divide the ball into two groups of cells, it will do so today. One group of cells will form the baby, and the other will form the baby's support system. The fluid-filled cell ball rests on the surface of your uterus. The cell ball now contains several hundred cells.

When the cell ball comes to rest on the surface of your uterus, the process of implantation begins. During implantation, the cell ball attaches to the surface of your uterus so it can receive protection and needed oxygen and nutrients from your bloodstream.

For Your Health A nutritious diet benefits your health and your baby's development.

Food Facts Steaming is the best and most convenient method for conserving nutrients in all types of vegetables.

DAY **7**	DATE:
	259 days to go

Implantation continues. The actual size of the implanted cell ball is .004 of an inch (0.1 mm).

When implantation is taking place, the cell ball actually burrows into your uterine lining, displacing some of its tissue. As a result, you may notice some light spotting.

Did You Know? Ten cell balls could fit into the space occupied by this printed period: .

IMPORTANT In hindsight, don't mistake this spotting for a light menstrual period. It's just the evidence that your pregnancy has begun.

notes

....

....

....

....

....

....

....

....

....

How are you feeling today?

MOOD: ....

ENERGY: ....

APPETITE: ....

MORNING SICKNESS? ....

CRAVINGS? ....

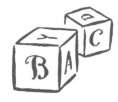

It goes without saying that you should never have more children than you have car windows.

ERMA BOMBECK

week 2

DAY
8
DATE:
258 days to go

During this week, the implanted cell ball will grow very rapidly. When implantation takes place, the organism is called an embryo.

Congratulations! You (actually your body) have finally officially met your developing baby. The two of you are now intimately joined, and your body begins to mobilize to support the baby's growth.

Did You Know? You don't realize it yet, but you've been pregnant for a whole week.

DAY
9
DATE:
257 days to go

Implantation is now complete. The embryo has actually sunk beneath the surface of the lining of your uterus. Growth is very rapid now: the amniotic sac (the bag of waters) and the amniotic cavity (the area within the womb that contains the amniotic sac, amniotic fluid, and developing child) have begun to form. The yolk sac will appear (this structure will give rise to the baby's digestive tract). These structures require the next six days to complete their formation.

You may notice some more light spotting as the implantation process is completed.

IMPORTANT Even if you anticipate pregnancy, it's too early for a pregnancy test to be reliably accurate.

DAY
10
DATE:
256 days to go

Your embryonic baby continues to grow rapidly. The amniotic sac, amniotic cavity, and yolk sac are developing.

Good personal health habits have never been as important as they are now. If you are the type of person who already eats well-balanced meals, exercises moderately, gets sufficient rest, and does not drink alcohol or take drugs, stay the course. If you need an excuse to take better care of yourself, let your baby be that excuse. Any positive change at any time during the pregnancy benefits both you and the baby.

Did You Know? The embryonic baby is a self-contained unit that plays a role in creating its own environment. For example, its delicate tissues must be constantly bathed in fluids or they would dry out or be crushed. Your body anticipates this need. Even before the embryo is formed, some cells gather to make a transparent bubble. Fluid seeps into the bubble from surrounding maternal tissues, and the bubble becomes the amniotic sac containing amniotic fluid. (The word *amnion* is from a Greek word meaning "little lamb" because lambs are often born surrounded by their prenatal "bubble" or amniotic membrane.)

A baby is God's opinion that life should go on.
CARL SANDBURG

DAY 11	DATE:
	255 days to go

The amniotic sac, amniotic cavity, and yolk sac continue to form. The placenta begins to form at the site of implantation. Blood from your system starts to circulate within the placenta.

The hormone level within your body will rise dramatically during pregnancy. Some women experience nausea as their bodies adjust to the increase in pregnancy-supporting hormones (estrogen, progesterone, and hCG).

For Your Information The first system to function in your developing baby is its cardiovascular system (heart and blood vessels). Your baby's heart will be beating before your period is one week late.

Food Facts The calcification of the fetal skeleton will begin about six weeks from now. Calcium and phosphorus are needed for the composition of the baby's bones and teeth, so be sure to eat lots of dairy products or green, leafy vegetables and animal protein or take a phosphorus supplement.

You may begin to experience some nausea at this point. Fatigue, stress, and a prepregnancy diet low in vitamins, minerals, and carbohydrates can make your nausea more severe. Small, frequent meals are better than large, infrequent ones (pregnant women tend to feel better if their stomachs are neither too full nor too empty).

Did You Know? The event called fertilization or conception, involving the union of the human egg and sperm, was first scientifically observed in 1944.

notes

....

....

....

....

....

....

....

....

....

....

DAY 12	DATE:
	254 days to go

The amniotic sac, amniotic cavity, and yolk sac are well along in their development (the fourth day of their six-day growth period). The sac is called a yolk sac even though it contains no yolk and no nutrients. Your embryonic baby measures between .006 and .008 of an inch in length (0.15–0.20 mm). Five embryos could fit into the space occupied by this printed period: .

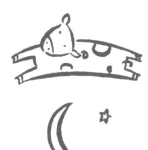

The surest way to make it hard for your children is to make it soft for them.

WESLEYAN METHODIST PROVERB

DAY	DATE:
13	*253 days to go*

Growth of the embryo continues to be rapid. Over the next two days, the chorionic villi appear (this is the tissue that lines the placenta). It is also the tissue that may be sampled if a chorionic villi sampling (CVS) is performed. CVS is a diagnostic procedure used to assess the baby's health and well-being in the first trimester.

If you need to settle your stomach, snack on dry crackers, toast, peppermints, or high-carbohydrate foods (like baked potatoes, vegetables, cereals, whole-grain breads, and dried beans and peas). Drink plenty of liquid. Avoid medications and food odors that make you feel queasy.

For Your Information Within this first month, the baby gathers nourishment from the mother through the hundreds of rootlike tufts that cover the amniotic sac. The food is channeled from the "roots" to the baby through a stalk that is the primitive umbilical cord.

Childbirth Then and Now In the second century A.D., the Greek physician Galen proposed a theory of prenatal development called *emboitement,* from a word meaning encasement, or encapsulation. He thought that tiny, preformed embryos existed in the "female semen" and that contact with the male merely brought about an "unshelling" of the embryo, permitting it to increase in size until birth.

DAY	DATE:
14	*252 days to go*

The chorionic villi are now fully formed. The amniotic sac, amniotic cavity, and yolk sac have also completed their development.

You may find that you are more tired than usual. Your body needs extra rest now because of all the internal activity connected with your pregnancy.

Did You Know? You still may not realize it, but by the time you go to bed tonight, you will have been pregnant for two weeks!

Food Facts Take steps to safeguard your health and the health of your baby. Don't eat uncooked eggs or cook with eggs that were cracked when you got them. Bacteria (such as salmonella, which causes food poisoning) can seep into the crack and penetrate the internal membrane of the egg.

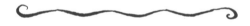

How are you feeling today?

MOOD: ....

ENERGY: ....

APPETITE: ....

MORNING SICKNESS? ....

CRAVINGS? ....

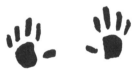

Your children are not your children. They are the sons and daughters of Life's longing for itself.
KAHLIL GIBRAN

week 3

DAY 15	DATE:
	251 days to go

The "primitive streak" appears (this is the forerunner of the brain and spinal cord). It is now possible to identify the head and tail sections of the baby's body.

By the end of this third week, you'll probably miss your menstrual period for the first time. You can celebrate your suspicions with a bottle of sparkling apple juice, grape juice, or ginger ale. Alcoholic beverages, no matter how diluted can cause birth defects and should not be drunk while you are pregnant.

IMPORTANT Prenatal alcohol exposure is the number one cause of mental retardation among newborns in the United States. Your baby needs all the advantages you can offer. Right now, exposure to alcohol would be a major disadvantage with potential complications. If you find it difficult to go without, try substituting alcohol-free beer or wine.

Did You Know? The amniotic sac or bag of waters that surrounds your baby is composed of two layers. The inner membrane is called the amnion, and the outer membrane is called the chorion. The chorion contributes tissue to help form the placenta.

Chart your waist size and weight here.

WAIST SIZE   WEIGHT

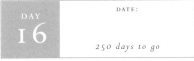

DAY 16	DATE:
	250 days to go

A groove is forming within the primitive streak through which cells will migrate to form three layers of tissue: the endoderm, the mesoderm, and the ectoderm. All of the baby's cells and organs will form from these three tissue layers. The bottom layer of cells (endoderm) forms the glands, lining of the lungs, tongue, tonsils, urethra and associated glands, bladder, and digestive tract. The middle layer of cells (mesoderm) forms the muscles, bones, lymphatic tissue, spleen, blood cells, heart, lungs, and reproductive and excretory systems. The top layer of cells (ectoderm) forms the skin, nails, hair, lens of the eye, lining of the internal and external ear, nose, sinuses, mouth, anus, tooth enamel, pituitary gland, mammary glands, and all parts of the nervous system. In addition, the cells from the middle layer will migrate to form a woven support for the developing organs. Another group of cells form clumps called "blood islands," which begin to form the baby's first blood cells. The genetic blueprint in each cell tells the cell what to do and orders its migration to the spot in the baby's body where the development will take place. It's a truly amazing process.

When I approach a child, he inspires in me two sentiments:
tenderness for what he is, and respect for what he may become.

LOUIS PASTEUR

While your pregnancy began with conception, your emotional experience of pregnancy started the first time you thought about having a baby and then decided to get pregnant. You might want to reflect on how you arrived at your decision to become pregnant. Was it an easy or a difficult decision? How long have you been thinking about becoming a parent?

For Your Information The true placenta does not begin to form until this week of development. The placenta forms at the site where the fertilized egg attached to the uterine wall. The chorionic villi are the fetal portion of the future placenta.

Food Facts Boiling is not recommended for cooking vegetables, because most of the nutrients are cooked out into the water. If you do prefer boiled vegetables to steamed during pregnancy, boil with just enough water to prevent burning (about ¼ cup).

notes

....
....
....
....
....
....
....
....
....
....
....
....
....
....

DAY 17	DATE:
	249 days to go

Another group of cells is migrating to the baby's head to form the "notochord," which gives rise to the vertebrae, or the bones of the spine. The cells in the notochord release a chemical that causes a dramatic change in the size of the cells in the ectoderm. These top-layer cells grow rapidly and form a thickened area called the neural plate, which will develop in the next few days.

You may notice that you feel more tired now than you normally do. Listen to your body and take that nap, sleep in if you can, and go to bed early.

Did You Know? Your baby is now .02 inch long (0.4 mm). Two or three babies the size of yours could fit into the space occupied by this printed period: .

DAY 18	DATE:
	248 days to go

Besides forming the baby's first blood cells, the cells that create the blood islands also form channels called the heart tubes. The heart tubes are fusing together—the first step in forming the baby's primitive heart, which will circulate the blood cells throughout the baby's body.

Most changes that accompany pregnancy are normal and although they may be uncomfortable are no cause for alarm. However, some symptoms need to be reported as soon as they occur so your practitioner can determine their importance.

Children seldom misquote you. They more often repeat word for word what you shouldn't have said.
MAE MALOO

Be sure to contact your practitioner if you experience: vaginal bleeding, menstrual-like cramps, or lower abdominal pain.

Food Facts Carrots are an excellent source of vitamin A during pregnancy. The vitamin A contained in carrots can be made more accessible to your body by cooking, chopping, grating, or juicing them.

DAY **19**	DATE:
	247 days to go

The fold of tissue that will form the baby's head can now be identified. The baby's body is beginning to unfold. The baby measures between .04 and .06 inch (1.0–1.5 mm) from head to tail.

Breast changes can be expected as your pregnancy continues. Tingling sensations and some soreness can be felt in your breasts during this early part of pregnancy.

For Your Health It's possible to detect your pregnancy with a pregnancy test now that you're this far along. Both the blood and the urine carry hCG, the hormone that is released into your system at implantation. All current pregnancy tests assess the presence of hCG to confirm pregnancy. A blood test is more sensitive than a urine test and can detect smaller quantities of hCG, but it still takes eight to nine days after implantation to build up detectable levels. A blood or urine pregnancy test can be performed in your practitioner's office or at a clinic. All home pregnancy kits test urine.

Food Facts Prepared foods should be eaten with caution during pregnancy. A label saying "All Meat" on a hot dog package does not mean the product is nothing but meat. According to the USDA, most franks contain 10% added water and 5% other ingredients, including flavorings and chemicals.

notes

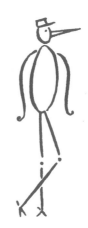

What's done to children, they will do to society.

KARL MENNINGER

DAY	DATE:
20	*246 days to go*

The next thirty days mark a critical period in the development of your baby's heart. While the heart itself consists of just two heart tubes, it has been joined to blood vessels in the baby's system. The next ten days mark a critical period in the development of the central nervous system. The mesoderm is now dividing into matched pairs on either side of the spinal column. These matched pairs of tissue called "somites" will eventually form the bones and muscles of your baby's head and body. Today, the first pair of somites will appear and thirty-eight pairs of somites will form between now and Day 30. The thyroid gland, eventually located at the base of the neck on either side of the windpipe, is also beginning to form. Today was a big day in the development of your baby's muscles, bones, and heart.

"Critical periods" are so named because they represent times during which the baby's organs and systems are growing most rapidly. Your health-conscious behavior can support these growth-spurt periods.

Did You Know? By this time, the amniotic sac is about the size of a grape.

DAY	DATE:
21	*245 days to go*

Four primitive chambers are forming in the baby's heart. Three pairs of somites are now present along the spinal column. The cavities of the chest and abdomen are forming. The baby now measures about ⅛ inch (1.5–2.5 mm).

Try as you might, you can't yet detect the baby's heartbeat without a special listening device. The function of this tiny heart is identical to its mature counterpart: to move around the oxygen and nutrient-rich blood cells that will feed the baby's developing tissues.

Did You Know? Today marks an important milestone in your pregnancy: either today or tomorrow, your baby's heart will begin to beat!

For Your Information The baby now looks like a tiny lump in the wall of your uterus. The entire "lump" extends out from the uterine wall about ⅓ inch (6.4 mm).

How are you feeling today?

Mood: ....

Energy: ....

Appetite: ....

Morning sickness? ....

Cravings? ....

Pregnancy defined is: Getting company inside one's skin.
Maggie Scarf

Week 4

DAY 22	DATE: 244 days to go

Between Week 4 and Week 8, the development of the baby's facial features takes place. Five folds of tissue accumulate at the base of the head to provide the raw material for the chin, cheeks, upper jaw, and ears. Two arches form that will become the upper and lower jaws. The groove of tissue that will form the larynx (voice box) and trachea (windpipe) appears. Five more pairs of somites have formed. Now eight pairs of somites are present, and the neural tube (later called the spinal cord) will begin to form between them. The chest and abdominal cavities are continuing to form. Lung buds (tissue from which the lungs will form) appear in the chest cavity. If the baby's heart didn't begin to beat yesterday, it will start today. Circulation is beginning to develop in the mesoderm, the yolk sac, and in the lining of the placenta.

Although you've been waiting for your period to start, by now you probably have an idea that you might be pregnant. A pregnancy test is always a good place to begin. Either check in with your clinic or physician or purchase a home pregnancy test kit. After a positive test, decide on a practitioner (see page 21) and schedule your first prenatal visit.

Did You Know? By the fourth week, the placenta begins to function as a means of nutrient, oxygen, and waste exchange between the mother and the baby.

For Your Information The baby's body measures about ¼ inch (6.4 mm) long (the size of a split pea). The heart (a U-shaped tube at this point) is only .1 of an inch (2 mm) long when it begins to beat. This seems tiny, but in proportion to the baby's body, the baby's heart is nine times as large as an adult's heart.

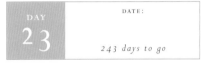

DAY 23	DATE: 243 days to go

The development that began yesterday continues today: the baby's jaws are appearing, the lung buds are forming, circulation is being established in the mesoderm and yolk sac, the lining of the placenta is developing, and the somites are forming. While the baby's physical appearance changes, its size changes, too—it gets bigger each day.

While you may be craving certain foods, you may also find that some things you eat may disagree with you. Heartburn, indigestion, bloating, and intestinal gas are not uncommon during pregnancy.

For Your Comfort
Take note of the foods that tend to cause you digestive problems and avoid them as much as possible until you feel more stable.

Did You Know? By the end of this month, your baby will have completed a period of growth that involves the greatest size and physical changes of its lifetime. In five days, it will be 10,000 times larger than the fertilized egg.

Kids are confused. Half of the adults tell him to find himself; the other half tell him to get lost.
WALTER MACPEEK

DAY **24**	DATE: *242 days to go*

The next eighteen days mark a critical period for arm and leg development. At this point, the baby has no visible arms or legs. But in another forty-eight hours, the tiny buds that will form the arms will suddenly appear. The eyes will also begin to form. The spinal cord is beginning to form between pairs of somites. Thirteen pairs of somites are now present. Liver and pancreas buds are present. The embryo now assumes a curved shape, with a prominent bump representing the head.

You may have noticed that you're experiencing some of the same emotions that often preceed menstruation: moodiness, irritability, tearfulness. While some of these feelings may have a psychological basis, most of the time they are just natural reactions to your body's changing levels of hormones.

Food Facts The nutritional value of food is the most important aspect of your diet during pregnancy. Green leafy vegetables are an important source of riboflavin, vitamin C, and iron, essential elements for mother and baby.

Did You Know? Proteins provide amino acids, which are required to build the baby's tissues. Seventy-four to 78 grams of protein are required each day during pregnancy. Milk, eggs, meat, fish, grains, cereals, legumes, leafy vegetables, and cheese are excellent sources of protein. For the nonvegetarian, two 2-ounce servings of animal protein and two servings of vegetables (especially legumes) should meet or exceed the daily requirement. The vegetarian can plan a menu that provides for her body's protein needs by including peanut protein + wheat, oats, rice, corn, or coconut; soy protein + corn, wheat, rye, or sesame; legumes + cereals; and leafy vegetables + cereals.

notes

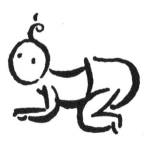

Childbirth is more admirable than conquest, more amazing than self-defense, and as courageous as either one.
Gloria Steinem

DAY 25	DATE:
	241 days to go

The eyes are beginning to form, and a tiny depression (or dimple) now marks the place on either side of the head where the baby's ear canal and inner ear will form. The digestive system is beginning to form from a portion of the yolk sac. In the next three days, the arm buds will appear.

You may begin to notice a need to urinate more frequently. This is normal and caused by pressure on your bladder from your growing uterus along with an improved metabolism that helps your body eliminate waste more quickly. Your breasts may feel fuller, heavier, and tender. You may also notice the areola, or pigmented portion of your breast, darkening somewhat.

This week marks a critical period in the development of your baby's gastrointestinal tract.

Childbirth Then and Now In 1639, author Owen Woods in *An Alphabetical Book of Physical Secrets* suggested a pregnancy test: if a woman saw her reflection in her boiled urine, she was pregnant.

DAY 26	DATE:
	240 days to go

The aorta of the baby's heart is beginning to form. The aorta is the largest artery of the body, carrying blood away from the heart to all organs and tissues. The baby's length is now measured from the top of its head (crown) to the bottom of its bottom (rump). The "crown-to-rump" length at Day 26 is between .11 and .20 inches (3–5 mm).

Selecting a practitioner is an extremely important task. You need to weigh many considerations as you choose the person who will direct the medical course of your pregnancy and attend the birth of your baby. Before deciding on a practitioner, you should ask them about their philosophy of childbirth: Will they consult with you? Do they routinely do episiotomies? Will they attend a homebirth if that is an option? and so on.

For Your Health Maintaining a normal red blood cell count is dependent on an adequate intake of protein.

Did You Know? The baby's tiny heart pumps sixty-five times a minute to circulate the newly formed blood and nourish developing tissues.

DAY 27	DATE:
	239 days to go

By now the arm buds have appeared and a tiny liver has formed. The liver has many important functions involving the utilization of nutrients: it stores excess blood sugar and releases it when required, stores and metabolizes fat, breaks down excess protein (amino acids), synthesizes blood-clotting factors, and breaks down (or detoxifies) poisonous substances, including alcohol. The gall bladder, stomach, intestines, pancreas, and lungs are beginning to form. The thyroid continues its development.

Your first prenatal visit involves a complete physical examination, an assessment of pregnancy symptoms, a number of laboratory tests such as tests for sexually transmitted diseases, cervical cancer, anemia, and other conditions, as well as

Children can forgive their parents for being wrong, but weakness sends them elsewhere for strength.
LEONTINE YOUNG

protection against rubella and blood type—and the compiling of a complete medical and health history.

IMPORTANT Be sure to remember the first day of your last menstrual period. That date will come in handy when your practitioner estimates your due date.

Food Facts Extreme weight gain during pregnancy may be due to an excessive intake of sugar, especially from foods such as desserts, muffins, jam, ice cream, candy, and chocolate.

notes

....

....

....

....

....

....

....

....

....

....

....

....

....

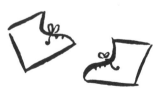

DAY 28	DATE:
	238 days to go

The lenses of the baby's eyes are beginning to form. The lens bends the light that enters the eye to focus a clear image for vision. The arms now look like flippers. In the next three days, the leg buds will appear. The first of three sets of kidneys appear. (This set never becomes functional, however.) The baby is shaped like a C, and the prominent feature is the tail, or end portion, of the baby's body, which now measures .16 to .24 inches long (4–6 mm) crown to rump.

Today marks the end of the first month of your pregnancy (each gestational month is based on a lunar month of twenty-eight days or four seven-day weeks). Only eight and one half more months to go!

Did You Know? Kidneys are not necessary for your baby's growth and development before birth because the placenta is the major organ of fetal excretion.

Food Facts Hot cereals made from unrefined grains (like oats, wheat and corn) are valuable sources of B vitamins and in combination with milk offer high-quality protein during pregnancy.

How are you feeling today?

MOOD: ....

ENERGY: ....

APPETITE: ....

MORNING SICKNESS? ....

CRAVINGS? ....

Each child is an adventure into a better life, an opportunity to change the old pattern and make it new.
HUBERT H. HUMPHREY

Lunar Month 2

Include sufficient folic acid in your diet to support the development of your baby's brain and nervous system.

Drink at least 8 glasses (64 fluid ounces) of water every day and maintain your well-balanced diet.

Exercise to strengthen the muscles of your pelvic floor and to improve your general health.

Moisturize dry skin; keep oily skin clean.

Prevent varicose veins or minimize their symptoms.

Include sufficient B5, B12, folic acid, and iron to support the increased volume of blood being produced by your system.

Prevent breast sagging by wearing a supportive bra and exercising your chest muscles.

Get plenty of rest.

Eat a light snack before bedtime and increase sugar intake to prevent morning sickness.

Remain drug- and alcohol-free and limit daily caffeine intake.

week 5

Chart your waist size and weight here.

WAIST SIZE   WEIGHT

The lenses of the baby's eyes continue to form. The surface layer of the baby's skin will be formed during this month. The tongue is recognizable and the nasal pits are beginning to form. The lymphatic system (the system that filters out bacteria and other foreign particles) is beginning to develop. A second nonfunctional set of kidneys appears. The arms still look like flippers. The gonads are present but have not developed into ovaries (if your baby is a girl) or testes (if your baby is a boy). In eight more days (by Day 37), the baby will be twice as long as it is today.

During the next six days, the baby's brain, body, and head will undergo a period of rapid growth. Do all you can to support this growth. Folic acid is of particular importance to the development of the brain and nervous system. Folic acid (along with other vitamins and coenzymes) is also responsible for the normal development of blood cells within the baby's bone marrow. Green leafy vegetables and walnuts are natural sources of folic acid. Talk to your practitioner about the pros and cons of a vitamin and mineral or folic acid supplement.

Did You Know? Leg development always lags slightly behind arm development until the third year of the baby's life.

Food Facts Good nutrition is the most important aspect of a healthy pregnancy.

| DAY 30 | DATE: |
| 236 days to go | |

By this time, thirty-eight pairs of somites have formed (the somites form the bones and muscles of the head and trunk). If they haven't appeared already, the leg buds will be present today. The baby's brain has differentiated into the three main parts possessed by all human brains: the forebrain, the midbrain, and the hindbrain. The hindbrain contains regions that help regulate heart rate and breathing and coordinate muscle movements; the midbrain is a relay station, sending messages to their final destinations in the brain; and the forebrain has specialized structures called "lobes" that translate input from the senses, play a role in memory formation and storage, and engage in "higher order" processing, like thinking, reasoning, and problem solving. The baby now measures ¼ inch (6–7 mm) long—that's 10,000 times bigger than at conception in only thirty days.

An ultrasound test (sonogram) can be performed any time from this point (Week 5) on. Your practitioner will discuss the rationale behind any prenatal diagnostic procedures ordered.

There are only two things a child will share willingly—communicable diseases and his mother's age.
DR. BENJAMIN SPOCK

Did You Know? The yolk sac that developed early in the first month is now dysfunctional and will diminish in size. It remains a tiny lump of useless tissue until birth, when it is expelled as part of the afterbirth.

Food Facts Eggs are a balanced source of all important vitamins (except vitamin C) and minerals, and each egg offers 6 g of high-quality protein.

DAY **31**	DATE:
	235 days to go

Rapid brain and head growth continues. Cups are formed that will contain the eyeballs. A primitive mouth appears. The groove of tissue that appeared on Day 22 will now separate from the trachea (windpipe) and develop into the esophagus (the tube through which food is swallowed).

Most women don't notice much change in their own bodies yet. When you first start to show your pregnancy, you'll start to bulge in your lower abdomen beneath your belly button. That's where your uterus is situated.

For Your Information By the end of this month, the embryo will look like a tiny baby.

Food Facts Soybeans are the only food in the vegetable kingdom that contains all the essential amino acids the body needs to synthesize protein. The development of the baby's brain cells is particularly dependent on available protein.

DAY **32**	DATE:
	234 days to go

The baby's arms now look less like flippers and more like paddles.

The baby's development requires lots of fluids: remember that it is floating in amniotic fluid, which is constantly being replaced. For this reason and for the more efficient removal of waste, drink plenty of liquids.

For Your Health Water is the best hydrator. Drink at least 8 glasses (64 fluid ounces) every day.

Food Facts Milk is an excellent source of protein, calcium, phosphorus, vitamin A, and vitamin D. During pregnancy your body needs 400 IU of vitamin D daily to promote the absorption of calcium by your intestine. Skim milk and low-fat milk are probably the best choices during pregnancy to avoid fat and calories. Whole milk can contribute to high cholesterol for adults.

notes

....

....

....

....

....

....

....

....

....

....

....

....

Once you bring life into this world, you must protect it. We must protect it by changing the world.
ELIE WEISEL

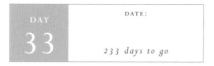

DAY

3 3

DATE:

233 days to go

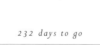 The nasal pits are now prominent. The developing heart can be seen through the baby's chest wall. The final (and permanent) set of kidneys has been formed. In about a week, the kidneys will produce urine. In the next four days, the hand plates will appear (each hand plate contains the tissues that will form the hands and fingers). The baby now measures about ⅓ of an inch (7–9 mm) in length.

If you're still feeling a bit queasy around food or after you eat, avoid rich, spicy, or creamy foods and strong smells, such as cigarette smoke and fried foods. It might also help if you eat more starchy foods like potatoes and pastas.

Food Facts For energy, 700–800 IU (2–2.5 mg) of vitamin B_1 (thiamin) is needed daily during pregnancy. One-half cup of enriched rice or pasta fulfills almost 10% of your daily thiamin requirement.

DAY

34

DATE:

232 days to go

Because of the rapid brain growth that has been occurring, the baby's head is much larger than its trunk. The nasal pits are easily seen. The baby's legs now resemble paddles.

You will continue to feel more tired than usual. Rest when you're tired; try not to push yourself, since exhaustion comes more rapidly than before. If you're on a schedule and worried that you'll sleep too long, use an easy-to-set alarm clock.

Then you can relax, rest for ten to thirty minutes, and the alarm will wake you so you won't have to keep checking the time.

Food Facts Everyone needs some fat in their diet to maintain the health of their skin and hair, protect their body organs from extremes in internal temperatures, and provide an energy reserve when carbohydrates are unavailable or depleted. In the diets of many pregnant and nonpregnant women in the United States, however, too much fat is ingested. Fat makes up 80% of both butter and margarine, so "lite" or fat-free spreads should be investigated as substitutes if you are getting too much fat in your diet. Pastry, bacon, ice cream, and fried foods also contain significant amounts of fat.

How are you feeling today?

Mood:

Energy:

Appetite:

Morning sickness?

Cravings?

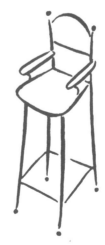

Kids really brighten a household. They never turn off the lights.
Ralph Bus

DAY	DATE:
35	231 days to go

notes

By now, the division between the cerebral hemispheres (two halves of the baby's brain) is well marked. The upper and lower jaws are present. Mammary gland tissue is beginning to develop in both females and males. The baby weighs about .00004 ounce (.001 g) (that's about as heavy as an eyelash from your lower lid).

Your ovaries don't ovulate during pregnancy. Many immature egg cells on the surface of the ovary temporarily develop, but never to the point of maturity because the appropriate level of hormonal stimulation is absent. Today marks the end of the fifth week of your pregnancy.

Did You Know? By this time, your embryonic baby displays a whole-body reflex in response to touch. This means that their developing nervous system is communicating with the primitive muscles and the muscles are beginning to contract in response to the nervous system's commands. Reflex-based neuro-muscular communication forms the foundation of all of your baby's behavior, both in your uterus and after birth.

Food Facts To help sustain growth, 1.6–1.7 mg of vitamin B_2 (riboflavin) is required daily during pregnancy. One cup of dark green leafy vegetables or one cup of skim milk or 2% milk supplies 25–30% of the minimum daily riboflavin requirements.

In their eagerness for their children to acquire skills and to succeed, parents may forget that youngsters need time to think, and privacy in which to do it.

JAMES COX

week 6

The cerebellum, the area of the brain that coordinates muscle movement, is beginning to develop. A primitive palate is forming on the roof of the baby's mouth. The baby's hand plates (flat rounds of tissue that will become the hands) will appear by today if they aren't already present. The elbow and wrist regions of the arm are becoming identifiable. The spleen (the organ that produces antibodies and removes worn-out red blood cells and bacteria from the bloodstream) is beginning to develop. The liver is now large enough to produce a bulge in the baby's abdomen.

You'll want to ask your practitioner about Kegel exercises to strengthen the muscles of your pelvic floor. When these muscles are properly toned, they will help carry the load of your heavy uterus as well as being more responsive during labor and delivery.

Food Facts Avoid breakfast meats during pregnancy. Pork sausage, bacon, and breakfast sausage may contain as much as 50% fat.

Childbirth in Other Cultures In ancient Japan, the umbilical cord was severed from the placenta after birth and wrapped in several thicknesses of white paper, with the outer covering containing the full names of the mother and the father. Once the child became an adult, the paper-wrapped cord was carried with them constantly.

The pituitary, or master gland, is beginning to form in the baby's brain. This gland produces growth hormone and other hormones that regulate the function of other glands, especially the thyroid, adrenal glands, and gonads (ovaries or testes). The olfactory bulb (connected with the sense of smell) is also beginning to form in the brain. During the next four days, pigment will begin to form in the retina of the eye and the lower limb paddles will develop foot plates. The windpipe (trachea), voice box (larynx), and bronchi (tubes that lead to the lungs) are beginning to form. The baby now measures .3 to .43 inch long (8–11 mm), having doubled in length in just eight short days.

From Week 1 to Week 15, the amniotic fluid volume increases at an average rate of one tablespoon plus two teaspoons (25 ml) per week.

Did You Know? Your baby is growing at a phenomenal rate. If your child grew as fast right after birth as it is growing right now, it would measure 15 feet tall by the time it was one month old.

Food Facts B vitamins, which include niacin, promote the normal, healthy functioning of all body systems. Your niacin intake during pregnancy will be adequate if your protein intake is adequate.

There is only one pretty child in the world, and every mother has it.
OLD ENGLISH PROVERB

DAY 38	DATE:
	228 days to go

Swellings are developing where the external ears will eventually be. The upper lip is beginning to form. The intestines are beginning to form within the umbilical cord. They will migrate into the abdomen when the baby's body is big enough to hold them. Primitive germ cells are arriving at the genital area. These cells will respond to genetic instructions to develop into either female or male structures.

No matter how happy you may be to be having a baby, you may experience a mild degree of irritability or depression during these early months of pregnancy because of the biochemical fluctuations that normally take place. Changes in neurotransmitter levels (the substances that allow nerve cells to communicate with each other) and hormones are primarily responsible.

Food Facts Vitamin B_{12} plays a role in protecting nerve fibers, promoting nervous system growth, and producing red blood cells. A daily intake of 4 mg of vitamin B_{12} is recommended during pregnancy. Anyone who eats meat, eggs, or milk products on a daily basis is guaranteed an adequate intake. Strict vegetarians can supplement their diets or drink vitamin B_{12} fortified soy milk.

Did You Know? As you read about your baby's progress, perhaps you've noticed that the arms develop before the legs, the upper lip forms before the lower lip, and the brain grows more sophisticated than the rest of the organs. There is a pattern here: it's called "cephalocaudal" development. Simply stated, for some cell clusters, growth proceeds from the head (cephalo) to the tail (caudal). Thus, organs and systems have to wait their respective turns, since some development is sequential rather than random or simultaneous.

notes

DAY 39	DATE:
	227 days to go

By tomorrow, the baby's lower limb paddles will have developed foot plates and pigment will be present in the retina of the baby's eye.

Your skin may start to break out or dry out. Complexion problems are due to an increased secretion of oils and to the hormonal changes of pregnancy.

For Your Comfort
Moisturize dry skin; keep oily skin clean by washing with a mild soap or face wash. Do not take acne medication. Ask your practitioner about the complicating effects of such medications.

Food Facts Chocolate and cocoa contain caffeine from the cocoa bean. If you cannot eliminate caffeine completely during pregnancy, at least cut back to less than two cups of coffee or its equivalent per day.

Pretty much all the honest truth telling there is in the world is done by children.
OLIVER WENDELL HOLMES

DAY 40	DATE: *226 days to go*

The palate continues to develop. The jaw and facial muscles are beginning to form. The baby teeth are developing beneath the baby's gums. The baby's heart begins its separation into four chambers. By this time the heart's energy output is 20% that of an adult. The diaphragm is forming as well (this is a piece of tissue that separates the chest cavity from the abdomen).

The metabolism of glucose may play a role in morning sickness. To make sure their glucose level doesn't fall too low by morning, pregnant women are advised to eat a light snack before going to bed (milk, toast, etc.). Extra sugar should be included; fried foods and foods high in fat should be avoided.

Did You Know? During these first forty days of development, your baby has grown .04 inch (1 mm) a day, but the growth rate is not even throughout its body: one day, growth may be concentrated in the arms, the next day, in the back, and so forth.

Food Facts Since the baby's teeth require calcium for their development, eat plenty of foods that contain calcium, like cheeses, sardines, and broccoli. If your system can tolerate it, drink milk instead of tea, coffee, or soda. If milk doesn't appeal to you, try substituting other calcium-rich foods and drink plenty of water.

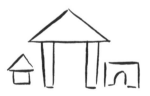

DAY 41	DATE: *225 days to go*

Because of all the rapid development, the baby's head is now much larger than its trunk. Over the next two days, the neck and trunk will begin to straighten (remember, prior to this point, the embryonic baby has been shaped like a C). Also, within the next two days, the hand plates will develop ridges indicating where the baby's fingers and thumb will be. As the process of forming the digital rays, or ridges, continues, the baby's hands will look like the shell of a scallop. The baby now measures nearly ½ inch long (11–14 mm). It is so small it would fit into a walnut shell and it weighs less than a book of matches.

Morning sickness is so named because it usually occurs immediately after getting up in the morning, but it can occur at any time of day. Generally, the symptoms (nausea and vomiting) disappear within a few hours.

Food Facts Vitamin B_6 is important in the metabolism of protein, and 2.5–2.6 mg are recommended during pregnancy. Meat, liver, vegetables, and whole-grain cereals are the richest natural sources of vitamin B_6. Vitamin B_6 can also be helpful in controlling the morning sickness that sometimes accompanies pregnancy.

Childbirth in Other Cultures Certain Filipino tribes believe that eating twin bananas can cause twins and that eating eggplant can cause a baby to be born with dark skin.

One of the obvious facts about grown-ups to a child is that they have forgotten what it is like to be a child.
RANDALL JARRELL

DAY **42**	DATE:
	224 days to go

 The digital rays, or ridges of the hand plates, should be completed today. Nipples are beginning to form for both sexes. Within the heart, the trunk of the pulmonary artery (the blood vessel that sends blood to the lungs to become oxygenated) separates from the trunk of the aorta. The baby's kidneys are beginning to produce urine. Today, the critical period for your baby's arm development has ended. The arms are now at their proper location and proportional size for this stage in development. The only task left is to complete the development of the hands.

By today, you may have missed your second menstrual period.

Did You Know? The cells in your uterus will increase between seventeen and forty times their nonpregnant size because they are being stimulated by extra amounts of estrogen (a hormone) and because of the stretching caused by the growing baby.

Food Facts To aid in the absorption of vitamin A, 10-15 mg of vitamin E is recommended daily during pregnancy. Vitamin E helps prevent the oxidation and breakdown of vitamin A and polyunsaturated fatty acids. About 60% of vitamin E in the diet comes directly from vegetable oil, margarine, salad dressing, and shortening. One tablespoon of any unsaturated oil (safflower, olive, canola [rapeseed], cottonseed, or corn) supplies at least 15 mg of the vitamin (100% of the daily requirement).

Chart your waist size and weight here.

WAIST SIZE WEIGHT

notes

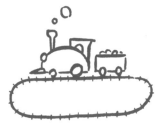

The Hebrew word for parents is horim, *and it comes from the same root as* moreh, *teacher. The parent is, and remains, the first and most important teacher that the child will ever have.*

RABBI KASSEL ABELSON

week 7

<table>
<tr><td>DAY</td><td>DATE:</td></tr>
<tr><td>43</td><td>223 days to go</td></tr>
</table>

Cartilage and bone are beginning to form in the baby's system. The ridges on the baby's hand plates are now well established. The gonads are forming and, over the next week or so, will become either testes or ovaries, depending on the sex of the baby. Over the next two days, indentations will form where the baby's knees and ankles will eventually develop.

Varicose veins are a common side effect of pregnancy. The extra volume of blood that your body produces to support the baby as well as the extra weight put pressure on the blood vessels in your legs.

For Your Comfort
Varicose veins can be prevented or their symptoms minimized by wearing support panty hose, elevating your legs when you are sitting, avoiding prolonged standing, avoiding excessive weight gain, and exercising (in moderation) thirty minutes a day.

How are you feeling today?

MOOD:

ENERGY:

APPETITE:

MORNING SICKNESS?

CRAVINGS?

<table>
<tr><td>DAY</td><td>DATE:</td></tr>
<tr><td>44</td><td>222 days to go</td></tr>
</table>

If any object touches the baby's head through the abdominal wall, the baby will turn away. Semicircular canals are beginning to form in the baby's inner ear that will sense balance and body position. The eyelids will begin to form over the next four days. The elbows will become visible in the next three days. By today, the indentations at the baby's knees and ankles are present. Over the next three days, the toe rays will appear. The critical period for the baby's leg development has ended. This means that the legs are now at their proper location and proportional size for this stage in development. Detail will be added (toes, joints, and toenails) in the time that remains.

If your skin generally breaks out before your period, you may be more likely to experience similar complexion problems now that you are pregnant.

Food Facts Calcium's most obvious role is in the formation of your baby's bones and teeth. Pregnant women require 1,200 mg of calcium daily. Milk and milk products are the richest sources: 1 cup of 2% milk offers 352 mg of calcium; 1 cup of skim milk, 296 mg; 1 cup of yogurt, 272 mg.

Did You Know? Today marks the day when the earliest recordable brain waves will occur.

Train up a child in the way he should go—and walk there yourself once in a while.
JOSH BILLINGS

DAY 45	DATE:
	221 days to go

In the next couple of days, the baby's nipples will become visible. During this week, your baby will begin to make spontaneous movements, as the connection improves between its brain and its tiny muscles and nerves. You won't be able to feel any of these movements yet, because the baby is still so small, rarely comes into contact with the uterine wall, and the motions involve little actual force. The baby now measures between ½ and ⅔ of an inch in length (13–17 mm).

Your blood volume level has been increasing gradually and will continue to do so. Your body actually produces more blood during pregnancy than it normally does so it can circulate blood to the embryonic baby and the pregnancy support structures (like the placenta) without interfering with your own blood needs.

For Your Health Your body needs vitamins B_6, B_{12}, folic acid, and iron to support the manufacture of red blood cells and plasma. Make sure you have sufficient amounts of these in your daily diet through supplements or by eating sufficient meat, vegetables, and whole-grain cereals.

DAY 46	DATE:
	220 days to go

The nasal openings and the tip of the baby's nose are formed. By today, the elbow region is clearly visible. Also, by today, the toe rays have appeared on each foot plate. The skin on the foot plate folds down between the future toes, distinguishing each from the other.

You will continue to notice breast changes: tingling sensations and tenderness. Your breasts may also feel fuller and heavier. Good breast support is crucial during pregnancy to prevent future sagging. Exercise to keep your chest muscles toned.

Food Facts About 5,000 IU of vitamin A are recommended during pregnancy. All yellow, orange, and dark green vegetables are rich in vitamin A (or carotene, an anticancer agent which is converted to vitamin A in the body).

notes

....
....
....
....
....
....
....
....
....
....
....

If there is a measure of good parenthood, it could be when your children exceed your own achievements.
Tom Haggai

DAY 47	DATE:
	219 days to go

By today, the baby's eyelids have begun to form. Over the next two days or so, the baby's basic body proportions will change: the trunk will begin to elongate and straighten.

As in previous weeks, you may continue to notice some heartburn and indigestion after you eat.

For Your Comfort
Try to stay away from foods that don't agree with you. It may be that during pregnancy some foods that you usually can tolerate will produce discomfort. Just take note of any changes, knowing that after pregnancy, the spicy food that you may crave now but can't eat will be just fine.

Food Facts Butter, milk, liver, egg yolk, and fish liver oils are also excellent sources of vitamin A.

DAY 48	DATE:
	218 days to go

The structure of the baby's eye is now well developed (it's not mature enough to do any visual processing yet, though). Over the next three days, the tongue will begin to develop. Distinct grooves are formed between the digital rays of the hands. The intestines are beginning to migrate from the umbilical cord (where they were originally formed) into the body cavity. The external ears are set low on the baby's head. As development proceeds, structures literally get pulled from one location to another. The baby's ears will not stay low-set (unless that is a family trait). They will be pulled to their normal position as the head grows in size and shape. Likewise, the eyes, although well-formed, are located on the sides of the baby's head, much like a rabbit, but they, too, will migrate forward as head development continues. The baby now measures between .62–.71 inches long (16–18 mm) and weighs about .033 ounce (0.94 g).

During this time, any diseases you have can be communicated to the embryo, so try to avoid exposure to communicable diseases. The most susceptible parts of the embryo are always those that are growing most rapidly at the time of the infection.

Did You Know? Between 1 teaspoon and ⅔ tablespoon (5–10 ml) of amniotic fluid is now present in your uterus.

For Your Information Even though your baby is surrounded by fluid, it does not drown because it does not depend on its lungs for air. Oxygen comes to the baby from you through the umbilical cord.

Parents learn a lot from their children about coping with life.
MURIEL SPARK

DAY 49	DATE: *217 days to go*

Over the next three days, the baby's arms will lengthen somewhat and begin bending at the elbow. The fingers and thumb have appeared, and are short and webbed with folds of skin in between.

When women don't plan their pregnancies, it may take them until about this time in the baby's growth to notice that they haven't had a period for about two months now and that something is going on. When you reflect back, you will see how much growth and change has taken place in your baby's system in only seven short weeks.

Did You Know? The baby's arms at this point are only as long as this printed 1.

For Your Information Human ovulation was first seen by scientists in 1930.

How are you feeling today?

MOOD:

ENERGY:

APPETITE:

MORNING SICKNESS?

CRAVINGS?

notes

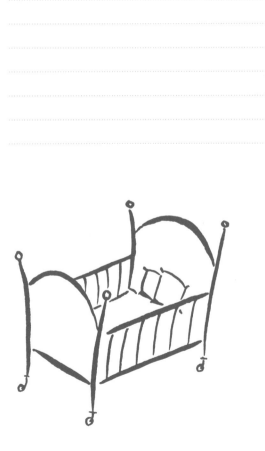

That most sensitive, most delicate of instruments: the mind of a little child.
HENRY HANDEL RICHARDSON

week 8

DAY	DATE:
50	*216 days to go*

DAY	DATE:
51	*215 days to go*

The surface of the baby's brain is now beginning to develop the rounds and fissures characteristic of humans. The upper lip is fully formed. Primary ossification centers are appearing in the long bones. These centers direct the replacement of cartilage by bone. The ossification process always starts in the upper arms, where the first true bone cells will replace the cartilage. If your baby is a girl, the clitoris is beginning to form (from the same tissue that the male penis will develop from). By this time, the critical period for the baby's heart development has ended. The heart will continue to grow and develop, but not at such a fast pace.

From Week 8 on, twelve to thirty small bumps called Montgomery's tubercles will appear on each areola. These tubercles are an enlargement of existing oil-bearing glands, and the oils they secrete will help keep your nipples soft and pliable.

For Your Information The baby's heart has been beating strongly. The stomach can produce some digestive juices, the liver can manufacture blood cells, and the kidneys can extract some waste products (uric acid) from the baby's blood.

Food Facts During pregnancy, take care to safeguard the nutritional value of the foods you eat. Baking a vegetable in its skin preserves most of its food value; microwaving vegetables with their skin on is likewise beneficial.

The retina of the eye is now fully pigmented. The baby's arms are longer and now bend at the elbow. The fingers and thumb are still short and webbed. Notches, or grooves, have formed between the toes on the foot plate. The baby's tail is still visible but is stubby.

You may begin to notice your clothing becoming tighter around the waist and bustline as your body changes and the baby grows. Are you showing yet?

Did You Know? The muscles of the baby's arms and body can already be "moved" by its brain.

Childbirth Then and Now In 1652, Philip Barrough in *The Method of Physick* recommended breathing through the pain of childbirth: "And if she was unskilled of pains of travell admonish her to hold and stop her breath strongly, and let her thrust it out to the flanks with all her might." During that time it was widely believed that birth pain could be eased if the woman would relax her pelvic region, a belief still strongly held today.

notes

....

....

....

....

....

....

A sweet child is the sweetest thing in nature.
CHARLES LAMB

DAY **52**	DATE:
	214 days to go

By today or tomorrow, the external ears will be completely developed. The bones of the palate are beginning to fuse and the taste buds are beginning to form on the surface of the baby's tongue. The feet are fan-shaped and the toes are webbed. The baby measures .71 – .79 inch (18–22 mm) from crown to rump.

The pigmentation changes that accompany pregnancy may become more noticeable by now. You may have noticed some blotchiness in your complexion and perhaps some darkening of the areola (the colored portion of your nipple). These changes are temporary and will disappear once the baby is born. By this time, the amniotic sac will be about the size of a chicken's egg.

For Your Information The appearance of the first bone cells in the baby's body marks the end of the embryonic period. This milestone was chosen since beginning bone formation coincides with the appearance of the basic structures and organs of the body.

Food Facts Potassium is critical to maintaining the heartbeat, preventing cellular dehydration, and facilitating nerve cell transmission and muscle contraction. A daily dose of 1,875–5,625 mg is considered safe and adequate. A potassium supplement is not advised, but bananas are an excellent source of potassium during pregnancy. Do not place bananas in the refrigerator until they are as ripe as you want them. The skin will turn brown in the refrigerator, but the fruit will remain unchanged.

DAY **53**	DATE:
	213 days to go

Today the baby measures between .87 and .94 inch (22–24 mm) in length, four times as long as it was just one month ago. If you experienced a comparable growth rate, within a month from now you would have to duck to stand in a room with a twenty-foot ceiling.

X-ray exposure should be avoided since the radiation can penetrate the embryo.

Food Facts Black tea is fermented to remove some of the tannin (a bitter-tasting acid in coffee and tea). Tannin and caffeine are kept to a minimum when tea is brewed quickly with freshly boiled water.

For Your Health Phosphorus is the mineral in second largest quantity in the body. It combines with calcium in the bones and is part of the structure of all body cells; 1,200 mg is recommended daily during pregnancy. Animal protein is one of the best sources of phosphorus. If your diet is adequate in calcium and protein, then it's adequate in phosphorus, too. However, too much phosphorus and too little calcium in your diet may be responsible for cramping.

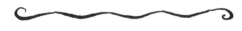

How are you feeling today?

MOOD:

ENERGY:

APPETITE:

MORNING SICKNESS?

CRAVINGS?

A torn jacket is soon mended; but hard words bruise the heart of a child.
HENRY WADSWORTH LONGFELLOW

DAY 54

DATE:

212 days to go

The baby's eyelids are more developed now, and the tongue is fully formed. Today, the external ears will complete their development. The baby's toes are unwebbed and appear longer.

The rapid rate of growth experienced by your baby over the past three to four weeks will continue and, at times, even quicken. Do all you can do to have the healthiest baby possible: be well rested, well nourished, well hydrated, well exercised, relaxed, and drug- and alcohol-free.

For Your Information The word *placenta* comes from the Greek for "flat cake."

Food Facts Herbal teas contain no caffeine and many are believed to have healing properties. If you normally drink caffeinated tea or coffee, you may want to substitute herbal tea during your pregnancy.

DAY 55

DATE:

211 days to go

Over the next two days, the male scrotum will begin to swell (the scrotum is an out-pocket of the abdominal wall that houses the testes). The baby is .91 to 1.10 inch (23–28 mm) long.

From this week on, there will be a 40–50% increase in your blood volume, mainly in the liquid portion of the blood (the plasma). There will be only a slight increase in your red blood cell count.

Did You Know? Under the direction of the genes, the baby's development proceeds like clockwork, with

each part geared to each other part. The two ears will develop in unison, for example. However, babies will have individually shaped ears, according to their family pattern.

DAY 56

DATE:

210 days to go

The head now looks rounded. The eyelids are beginning to unite, and the eyes appear half-closed. The fingers and toes are separated. By today, the thin layer of ectoderm that has covered the baby has been replaced by a layer of rather flattened cells, which will become the surface layer of the baby's skin. The intestines have begun their migration, but are still primarily located in the umbilical cord. The baby's sex still can't be identified by looking at the external genitals. The tail has disappeared. The baby measures 1 inch long (25.4 mm) and weighs about .04–.11 ounce (1–3 g).

When you go to bed tonight, you will have been pregnant for two months. Right now your uterus is about the size of a medium orange or a tennis ball. It's amazing that so much change can take place in a baby whose movements you can't even feel yet. In another two months or so, your baby will be big enough to make its motions felt. Then, in addition to the symptoms of your pregnancy, you'll have a closer encounter with your growing daughter or son.

For Your Information You are now carrying a well-proportioned, small-scale baby, no longer considered an embryo.

Did You Know? The baby's umbilical cord will grow to be about ¾ inch (19.1 mm) in diameter.

Children think not of what is past, nor what is to come, but enjoy the present time, which few of us do.
JEAN DE LA BRUYÈRE

Lunar Month 3

Continue to eat well, drink plenty of liquids, get plenty of rest, and urinate when you feel the need.

Get sufficient dietary iron to support blood volume changes and red blood cell development.

Continue your program of moderate exercise, but avoid jarring the uterus.

Take care not to gain excess body weight.

Avoid second-hand smoke; continue to be drug- and alcohol-free.

Avoid or minimize varicose veins, morning sickness, and constipation.

Minimize the likelihood of stretch marks by keeping your skin toned and weight gain gradual.

Avoid feeling faint or dizzy by changing position slowly, especially if you have been lying down, and forgo very hot baths, hot tubs, and spas.

Be aware that you might be able to feel the baby move just about anytime now.

Contact your practitioner if there are any changes in your normal vaginal secretions.

Don't take any medications (i.e., for headache, etc.) without your practitioner's approval.

week 9

DAY 57	DATE:
	209 days to go

 The baby's head now makes up more than half of its length. Over the next four days, fingernails, toenails, and hair follicles will appear (these are all specialized parts of the top layer of skin). Over the next week, the baby will assume a more upright posture. Week 9 is a period of rapid growth. Although the average rate of growth until birth is .06 inch (1.5 mm) in length per day, the baby will begin to grow even more rapidly from this point.

You may find your appetite increasing now that some of the nausea and discomfort have stabilized and the baby's growth is placing so many nutrient demands on your system.

Did You Know? From now until birth, the baby is technically called a "fetus." The word *fetus* comes from the Latin meaning "offspring."

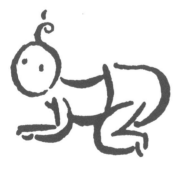

DAY 58	DATE:
	208 days to go

The baby's face looks rather wide and flat. The baby measures between 1 inch and 1.22 inches in length (27–31 mm).

As your blood volume increases, you may notice veins becoming more visible in your legs, breasts, and abdomen. Follow recommended guidelines, such as wearing support stockings, gaining no excess weight, elevating the feet, and exercising to improve blood flow, to prevent varicose veins in your legs or to minimize their symptoms.

Chart your waist size and weight here.

WAIST SIZE   WEIGHT

Food Facts Refined sugar is one of the most harmful "nonfoods" on the market. It contributes nothing to the body except calories and has been linked in some way to almost every major disease. In addition, it rots teeth! Refined sugar is found in brown sugar, white sugar, honey, maple syrup, and corn syrup. Alternatives to refined sugar include dried fruit and other foods that are naturally sweet-tasting. Artificial sweeteners can be used in moderation during pregnancy.

If you bungle raising your children, I don't think whatever else you do well matters very much.
JACQUELINE KENNEDY ONASSIS

DAY
59

DATE:

207 days to go

The baby's eyes are still set wide apart. This is only a temporary location until the head completes its development. The baby's body continues to straighten; its torso lengthens and its posture becomes more upright.

Your uterus is now about the size of a small grapefruit.

For Your Health Each day you need to include 80–100 mg of vitamin C in your diet. Vitamin C helps build connective tissue for the arteries, aids in the absorption of iron, and is an antioxidant. Excellent sources of vitamin C include fresh orange juice, bell peppers, fresh grapefruit juice, papaya, brussels sprouts, broccoli, and oranges.

Food Facts Fluid intake is important, but avoid soft drinks—they have approximately nine teaspoons of sugar for every 12-ounce serving.

DAY
60

DATE:

206 days to go

Over the next four days, the baby's skin will thicken and become less transparent.

Avoid second-hand smoke and exposure to other pollutants. Smoke and pollutants enter your lungs, are carried along with the oxygen by your bloodstream, and then are transmitted to your baby's system in the oxygen-exchange process. Make sure your home is well ventilated and that you operate within smoke-free environments outside your home.

Food Facts Chloride is an ion that combines with sodium to allow for the free movement of fluids within the cells and maintains the stomach's acidity. As an element, the liquid chlorine added to public drinking water helps to eliminate water-borne diseases like typhoid fever. Most Americans receive sufficient chloride through their drinking water. The chloride requirements are similar for pregnant and nonpregnant women.

For Your Information Water, vitamins, electrolytes (minerals like sodium, potassium, and chloride) and other minerals are needed for your baby's blood formation and growth, and for maintaining various body processes.

notes

....
....
....
....
....
....
....
....
....
....
....
....
....

You have to love your children unselfishly. That's hard, but it's the only way.
BARBARA BUSH

DAY	DATE:
61	205 days to go

The colored portion of the eye (the iris) will begin to develop over the next three days. Over the next two days, the eyelids will meet and temporarily fuse shut.

Consistent with pigmentation changes during pregnancy, you may notice that your moles, freckles, recent scars, or dark birthmarks are darkening along with your vagina, cervix, and vulva. This is quite predictable and temporary.

As adults grow older, they sometimes develop a reduced tolerance to milk and milk products. If that is the case with you, check with your practitioner for other sources of calcium and phosphorus.

Childbirth in Other Cultures In Sweden, all births take place in hospitals managed by highly trained midwives. Prenatal care is free and provided for every woman. Absence of prenatal care is unheard of.

notes

....
....
....
....
....
....
....
....
....

DAY	DATE:
62	204 days to go

Ossification centers are established in the skull; those in the long bones continue to develop as the baby becomes more solid. The baby's bones and muscles are growing rapidly. The baby's body begins to attain proportions more like a newborn baby's.

Although weight gain fluctuates from week to week, your average weight gain during this second trimester is about a pound a week.

Food Facts To support the baby's production of cartilage and bone tissue, four servings of calcium-containing foods will probably satisfy the 1,200 mg daily requirement. In addition to milk and yogurt, other excellent food sources of calcium include cheese (especially Swiss, Provolone, and Monterey Jack), sardines, salmon, and broccoli.

Childbirth in Other Cultures In northern Russia during the 1800s, the custom was for the midwife to require the laboring woman and her husband to give the names of the people, besides their spouse, with whom they had "cohabited" (slept with). If the labor was an easy one, both had told the truth; if the labor was difficult, either the wife or the husband had lied.

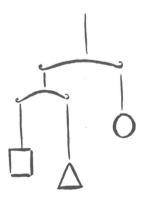

The illusions of childhood are necessary experiences: a child should not be denied a balloon because an adult knows that sooner or later it will burst.

Marcelene Cox

DAY **63**	DATE:
	203 days to go

The skin has become thicker and less transparent. The vagina is beginning to develop in females. The penis is now distinguishable in males. The baby has now attained a more upright posture. In one short week, your baby almost doubled its length to about 2 inches (51 mm) and more than doubled its weight, to about ¼ ounce (7.6 g).

Every baby shows a distinct individuality in behavior by the end of the third month. This is because the actual structure of the muscles varies slightly from baby to baby. The alignment of the muscles in the face, for example, follows an inherited pattern. The facial expressions of the baby are already similar to the facial expressions of the parents.

Food Facts Sodium is an element found in table salt. Along with potassium, sodium regulates the amount of fluid in the body and permits nerve cell transmission and muscle contraction. An intake of 1.1–3.3 g of sodium a day is considered safe and adequate. The highest concentrations in foods—thus, those to be avoided—are in cured ham, bacon, pickles, potato chips, and cold cuts, where the sodium is used as a preservative. Pregnant women should not normally restrict their sodium intake because of the extra demands placed on their body.

Childbirth Then and Now The first attempt to make newborn feedings follow a schedule was based on Dr. T. S. Southworth's observations in 1906. He recommended ten nursings a day for the first month, and eight a day in the second and third months. Today, nursing more frequently (eight to eighteen feedings per day in the first weeks) improves milk production and reduces nipple soreness.

notes

How are you feeling today?

MOOD:

ENERGY:

APPETITE:

MORNING SICKNESS?

CRAVINGS?

God could not be everywhere, and therefore he created mothers.
JEWISH PROVERB

week 10

<table>
<tr><td>DAY
64</td><td>DATE:

202 days to go</td></tr>
</table>

Sometime during the next three weeks, the urine that is formed by the baby's kidneys will be excreted into the amniotic fluid. The urine is sterile and is carried away in the regular replacement of the fluid.

You have probably gained 2-4 pounds by now. If you were underweight when you began your pregnancy, you will gain a little more than other women.

For Your Health Try to gain only needed weight by staying with your nutritious diet. Additional weight will add to your discomfort, increase your chances of getting stretch marks, and make it more difficult to lose weight after the baby is born.

Food Facts If you're hungry for ice cream and the product is called "French" ice cream, it means that there is a greater percentage of egg solids in the mixture. This means more protein, but also more cholesterol.

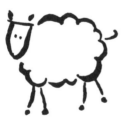

<table>
<tr><td>DAY
65</td><td>DATE:

201 days to go</td></tr>
</table>

Over the next three days, the baby's fingernails will begin to grow from the nail beds. The baby's skin is touch sensitive all over—any type of touch causes the baby to move.

About 90% of all women will develop stretch marks sometime during their pregnancy. If you have elastic, well-toned skin and try to keep weight gain steady and gradual, your chance of developing stretch marks will be reduced.

Did You Know? Good skin tone, good (nutrition to encourage) skin elasticity, and gradual (not rapid and not excessive) weight gain can prevent or minimize stretch marks. There are several lotions and creams on the market that boast results, but they don't really seem to help prevent anything but skin dryness, no matter what the manufacturer claims or how much you pay.

Food Facts Sulfur helps to stabilize protein structures in the body. Your skin, hair, and nails contain some of the body's most rigid protein and have a high sulfur content. Unfortunately, there is no recommended intake for sulfur, but you can aid your sulfur intake by eating dried apricots and prunes. Generally, sulfur deficiencies are unknown.

Don't be discouraged if your children reject your advice. Years later they will offer it to their own offspring.
OSCAR WILDE

DAY 66	DATE:
	200 days to go

The baby's brain now has the same structure it will have at birth, but it's not the same size it will be at birth. The thyroid, pancreas, and gall bladder will complete their development during the next three days.

With rare exceptions, you won't feel your lively baby move yet. The baby's newly formed muscles are weak, and the baby is so small that the womb has barely expanded and is still contained within the girdle of the hipbones.

Food Facts Meat is an excellent source of B vitamins and protein. Chopped sirloin makes the leanest ground meat, followed by ground chuck. To avoid health problems associated with undercooked ground meat, make sure all ground meat is well-done.

DAY 67	DATE:
	199 days to go

New reflexes are present: now when the baby's face is touched, it will open its mouth.

You may notice an occasional headache. Headaches during pregnancy are generally caused by hormonal changes, added stress, and increased sinus congestion. Vaginal secretions also respond to hormonal changes. Vaginal secretions become white and sometimes abundant during pregnancy. Report any changes to your practitioner.

 Don't take any medication without your practitioner's approval.

Childbirth in Other Cultures Women living in the Yucatán Peninsula give birth in the matrimonial hammock, the traditional bed of the couples of the region. The midwife is positioned on a low stool in front of the hammock.

notes

....

....

....

....

....

....

....

....

....

....

....

....

....

....

....

....

....

....

....

In the all-important world of family relations, three words are almost as powerful as the famous,
"I love you." They are "Maybe you're right."
 OREN ARNOLD

DAY 68	DATE:
	198 days to go

The baby's thyroid, pancreas, and gall bladder have now completed their development. Within the next three days the hard, bony part of the palate will be completely formed.

In addition to occasional headaches, you may notice some dizziness and faintness. If you are feeling light-headed, try to lie down and elevate your legs higher than your head. Get up slowly when you feel stabilized.

If you should faint, contact your practitioner. They'll want to know more about the cause.

Childbirth in Other Cultures Some tribal societies in New Guinea have no idea how long a pregnancy should last. They believe that a child could be born anytime the child decided to be, which leads to endless confusion. This means that if a man has been away from home for a year and a baby is born to his wife three months after his return, he does not question her fidelity. Instead, people believe the baby hurried up to see its father's face!

How are you feeling today?

MOOD:

ENERGY:

APPETITE:

MORNING SICKNESS?

CRAVINGS?

DAY 69	DATE:
	197 days to go

Over the next two days, the muscles in the walls of the baby's digestive tract will become functional in order to begin "practicing" the movements required to push food from one portion of the tract to another.

Despite occasional light-headedness, you may feel more emotionally stable now as your body gets more and more used to being pregnant. Every woman is different, however, and each pregnancy is unique, no matter how many children you have had.

Food Facts Pregnant women need at least 18 mg of iron each day. A woman's trace iron requirements increase dramatically during pregnancy to support the extra volume of blood and increases in red blood cell production. Liver, kidney, beef, eggs, whole-wheat bread, prunes, raisins, and green vegetables are all good sources of iron. In addition, an iron supplement is recommended during pregnancy.

Childbirth Then and Now The Greek physician Hippocrates devised a test he believed would reveal the sex of a developing child: if the woman's right breast was firmer, or her right eye brighter, she would have a boy; if the left breast was firmer or the left eye brighter, she would have a girl. Another ancient conviction was that boys sat higher in the womb than girls, a belief that has lasted well into the twentieth century.

Wouldn't it be wonderful to be as brilliant as our children thought we were when they were young, and only half as stupid as they think we are when they're teenagers?

DAISY BROWN

DAY 70	DATE:
	196 days to go

The hard, bony part of the baby's palate is now completely formed. This plate divides the mouth from the nose and makes it possible for the baby to eat and breathe simultaneously. The muscles in the walls of the digestive tract have become functional and are beginning to practice the contractions they will make when they have food to digest. The baby's growth rate has slowed somewhat. It has doubled its weight in the last week to almost ½ ounce (13 g); its length has increased to about 2 inches (50–61 mm).

Today marks the end of Week 10 of your pregnancy. Women are very apt to neglect treating morning sickness, but receiving medical advice sooner rather than later can help reduce the severity of the symptoms.

Did You Know? Cervix is the Latin word for "neck."

Food Facts Pure apple juice (with no sugar or preservatives) is an excellent beverage to drink during pregnancy. One cup of apple juice is a good source of iron, potassium, and magnesium.

notes

Small children disturb your sleep, big children your life.
YIDDISH PROVERB

week 11

DAY 71	DATE:
	195 days to go

Sometime during the next two weeks, the urine that is formed by the baby's kidneys will be excreted into the amniotic fluid.

Take care to wear comfortable clothes that don't restrict movement or inadvertently cut off your circulation. If you're not quite ready to wear maternity clothing yet, select transitional styles, such as loose sweaters and stretch leggings.

Chart your waist size and weight here.

WAIST SIZE   WEIGHT

Childbirth Then and Now In England from 1705 on, women were urged to have a healthy pregnancy by moderating their diets, sleeping as much as possible, and not wearing tight corsets. Cordials containing cinnamon, nutmeg, sugar, and eggs were served to warm and strengthen the mother-to-be.

Food Facts Dried fruits are an excellent source of iron during pregnancy, especially raisins (1 cup = 5.8 mg iron), apricots (1 cup = 8.2 mg), and peaches (1 cup = 9.6 mg). One cup of prune juice offers 10.5 mg of iron. The minimum daily iron requirement is 18 mg.

DAY 72	DATE:
	194 days to go

The baby's intestines are migrating from the umbilical cord to the abdomen.

Just as in the past two months, you will continue to feel more tired than usual. Continue to listen to your body and make adjustments in your schedule so you can rest when you need to.

Childbirth in Other Cultures Tsinghai women of China carry their babies with them for five years, nursing them on demand.

Food Facts If it agrees with you, cabbage is an excellent source of vitamin C. Serve cabbage raw in coleslaw, toss it along with other greens in salads, or stir-fry it in oil or butter (ten minutes until wilted) and sprinkle with sesame seeds for flavor. One-half cup of cabbage provides 24 mg of vitamin C or about a quarter of your daily requirement during pregnancy.

DAY 73	DATE:
	193 days to go

The placenta grows with the baby, but not as fast. At this point in development, it weighs around 1 ounce (28 g); at the time of birth, it will weigh between 1 and 2 pounds (448-896 g).

Morning sickness occurs in about 50% of pregnant women between Weeks 4 and 14. Most often, nausea is caused by the elevated hCG

If there must be trouble, let it be in my day, that my child may have peace.
THOMAS PAINE

levels in your bloodstream and your changed carbo-hydrate metabolism, but other conditions can also cause nausea and vomiting. Food may not be your friend yet, but most of the nausea should subside in another month or so.

TAKE NOTE If you experience food aversions, make sure you're not suffering any nutrient, vitamin, or mineral losses because you are avoiding certain foods or food groups.

Childbirth in Other Cultures In Holland, relaxation and relief of discomfort and pain during childbirth are managed entirely through breathing and relax-ation techniques. Medication is strongly discouraged. Today, the majority of women in Holland still give birth at home and their births are assisted by mid-wives, not physicians.

For Your Health Pregnancy makes women more prone to bladder infections, and the longer the urine stays in the bladder, the more likely it is to grow bacteria if such bacteria are present. Drink plenty of fluids to flush out your system; sufficient vitamin C intake and drinks high in acidity (like citrus and cranberry drinks) can help reduce your chances of getting a bladder infection.

Did You Know? Your baby will be born with 300 bones in its body. As your child grows, some bones will fuse together, to produce a total of 206 bones when it is an adult.

notes

DAY	DATE:
74	*192 days to go*

Over the next three days, the vocal cords will form in the baby's larynx, or voice box. The baby will not be able to make sounds, however, or cry out loud, because sound travels through air, not fluid.

You may continue to need to urinate frequently. Again, that's because your system is working more efficiently to remove waste and to circulate nutrients. It's important to empty your bladder when it feels full.

If we could learn how to utilize all the intelligence and patent good-will children are born with, instead of ignoring much of it—why—there might be enough to go around!

DOROTHY CANFIELD FISHER

	DATE:
DAY **75**	*191 days to go*

By today, all of the baby's twenty baby teeth and their sockets have formed in the gums. Over the next three days, the intestines will form into folds and become lined with villi (small, finger-like projections in the lining of the intestines that absorb certain nutrients).

Very hot baths during pregnancy may be exhausting and may cause fainting. Spas and hot tubs are to be avoided if the temperature is over 100°F.

Childbirth Then and Now The ancient Israelites considered new mothers "unclean" during the first few days after childbirth. The period of "uncleanliness" lasted for seven days after the birth of a boy, and fourteen days after the birth of a girl. The same idea was common among the ancient Greeks.

Food Facts Because Vitamin C is a water-soluble vitamin, it is not stored in the body's tissues and continually has to be resupplied. Practically all fresh vegetables are good sources of vitamin C during pregnancy, especially if eaten raw.

	DATE:
DAY **76**	*190 days to go*

By today, the baby's vocal cords will have formed in its larynx, or voice box.

A woman's carbohydrate intake (sugars, starches, and fiber) is usually more than adequate during pregnancy.

Food Facts Legumes (which include dried beans, peas, and lentils) are one of the best food values during pregnancy. They offer high-quality protein that is rich in iron, thiamin (B_1), and riboflavin (B_2). One cup of prepared dried beans or peas provides 15–20 mg of protein, about 25% of your daily requirement.

Childbirth in Other Cultures Among the Arapesh of New Guinea, fresh coconuts are reserved for tribal feasts and for women who are breastfeeding.

notes

And do respect the women of the world; remember you all had mothers.
ALLEN TOUSSAINT

| DAY 77 | DATE:
189 days to go |

notes

By this time, the baby's liver will have begun to secrete bile and the pancreas will have begun to produce insulin. The intestines have formed into folds and are lined with nutrient-extracting villi. Bile is produced by the liver but is stored in the gall bladder (already formed). (When there is food in the small intestine, the bile will be released into the intestine to help break down fatty foods for digestion.)

Just a word about your baby's developing digestive system. Right now the baby is receiving all its food preprocessed from you via the bloodstream, so there will be no food in the baby's digestive system until it starts to eat by mouth (rather than by umbilical cord).

Did You Know? Only 60% of American parents say they read to their children.

Food Facts Cold cereals are convenient and nutritious for snacks or breakfast during pregnancy. Low-sugar selections are best: crisped rice cereal and bran cereal with raisins contain less than 11% refined sugar; Grape Nuts contains less than 7% refined sugar; Corn Flakes and Corn Chex contain less than 8% refined sugar.

How are you feeling today?

MOOD:

ENERGY:

APPETITE:

MORNING SICKNESS?

CRAVINGS?

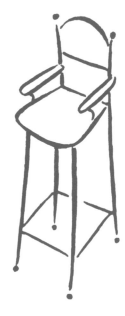

What war is to man, childbirth is to woman.

HINDU PROVERB

week 12

DAY **78**	DATE: _____ 188 days to go		**DAY** **79**	DATE: _____ 187 days to go	

The baby's hand is becoming more and more functional. The baby is beginning to use its thumb in opposition to the other fingers. Over the next three days, the external sex structures for both females and males will become clearly visible.

Once a woman becomes physically and emotionally adjusted to the impact of pregnancy, she generally enjoys a feeling of well-being—her appetite is good, and she looks and feels well. This well-being can only be experienced, however, if you are healthy, well nourished, and not overworked.

Childbirth Then and Now Many early agricultural societies believed that life was created when the sky or heaven (which was considered to be male) showered rain on the earth (considered to be female).

Food Facts In some regions, consumers have become sufficiently concerned about their local water supplies to turn to buying bottled water for personal consumption. The choice is an individual one, but all consumers should be alert to fraudulent claims. Mineral waters sold by European spas offer no known health advantages and may be undesirably high in sodium. Bottled water sold in the United States must be tested regularly for safety and must meet standards set by the Food and Drug Administration.

The baby practices inhaling and exhaling movements in the womb that send amniotic fluid in and out of its lungs. The presence of the fluid may be essential to the proper formation of the air sacs within the lungs.

By this time, you will probably have noticed some darkening of the area around the nipple (called the areola) and some enlargement of the areola's diameter.

Childbirth in Other Cultures In societies where men have never been allowed to witness childbirth, men fantasize about the terrible nature of birth. Arapesh men of New Guinea give pantomimed accounts of childbirth where women are depicted as writhing around in screaming agony. In reality, the Arapesh women give birth quietly and matter-of-factly on the damp ground of a steep slope in the dark with no one to help them but one other young woman. The new mother is expected to care for the newborn all by herself.

Food Facts The larger portions found in restaurants can be turned into small, frequent meals by asking for a take-home container as soon as you get your food and cutting portions in half. Eat half and take home the rest for a later time.

Neighbors' children are always the worst in the world.
GERMAN PROVERB

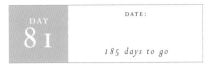

DAY 80	DATE: 186 days to go

The baby is now quite active, but is still so small it could easily move inside the egg of a goose.

Are you still experiencing bloating, indigestion, and heartburn after meals? Continue to watch what you eat, but try to eat smaller portions more frequently. One thing that happens during pregnancy is that the circular sphincter muscle that closes off the stomach from the esophagus relaxes and permits food and stomach acid back into the esophagus. The result is a burning sensation in the vicinity of your heart called heartburn (obviously, this sensation has nothing to do with your heart). If there is less food in your stomach, there is less to backwash into your esophagus, so you might feel more comfortable.

IMPORTANT Remember that your baby's hungry even though you might not be. Eat little meals frequently rather than skipping meals or eating only a couple large portions.

Food Facts Iodine is a trace element that is part of thyroxin, a hormone secreted by the thyroid gland that controls the way the body's cells use oxygen and release energy. A scant 175 mcg of iodine is recommended each day during pregnancy. The need for iodine is easily met by eating seafood and using iodized salt.

DAY 81	DATE: 185 days to go

Over the next three days, the baby's spleen will assume functions supervised by the liver: the removal of old red blood cells and the production of antibodies.

You may notice some constipation. As the pregnancy hormones relax the muscles of your bowel, elimination is made slower and less efficient. Also, your growing uterus presses on the bowel and further interferes with its activity.

For Your Health What to do about constipation? Exercise moderately, increase your fluid intake, and eat plenty of fruits and vegetables (preferably raw) to add fiber to your diet and help improve bowel function.

Food Facts Some cold cereals contain over 60% refined sugar. Of all cold cereals, Shredded Wheat contains the least amount of refined sugar (1–1.3%), followed by Cheerios, Puffed Rice, and Wheat Chex, which contain less than 3%.

notes

....
....
....
....
....
....
....
....
....

Never try to make your son or daughter another you; one is enough!
ARNOLD GLASOW

DAY 82	DATE:
	184 days to go

Much progress has taken place in the development of the baby's mouth. The bony palate, or roof of the mouth, has been complete for some weeks, the sucking muscles are filling out the cheeks, the tooth buds are present under the gums, the esophagus and windpipe are present, and the larynx, or voicebox, is present. By today, the baby's salivary glands will begin to function. Over the next three days, the baby will begin to make breathing, sucking, and swallowing motions.

By this time, most pregnant women can see a clear pattern of dilated veins on their chest and breasts.

Food Facts Bran cereals, whole-grain bread, peas, and baked beans are an excellent source of dietary fiber. Fiber helps the bowel function most efficiently and protects against bowel cancer. Fiber is particularly important during pregnancy, when constipation is common.

Childbirth in Other Cultures When Maori women of New Zealand give birth, they deliver on the ground near a stream. The Maori word *whenna* means both "earth" and "placenta."

DAY 83	DATE:
	183 days to go

By this time, the baby's heartbeat can be detected by a listening device called a Doppler. The spleen is now fully functional.

You've probably seen your practitioner two or even three times by now. Soon, the prenatal visits will become a predictable part of your routine. Make sure you take note of all the symptoms you are experiencing so your practitioner can determine their cause or impact on your pregnancy.

For Your Information During your pregnancy, your uterus will increase in weight from approximately 1 ounce (28 g) to more than 2¼ pounds (1120 g), more than 360 times its original weight.

Food Facts Zinc is a trace element that forms part of the structure of bone and is involved in DNA and protein synthesis, immune reactions, the action of insulin, and the utilization of vitamin A. The recommended daily intake of zinc during pregnancy is 20 mg. Animal foods are good sources of zinc, especially oysters, herring, milk, and egg yolks. Two small servings a day should provide sufficient zinc.

How are you feeling today?

MOOD:

ENERGY:

APPETITE:

MORNING SICKNESS?

CRAVINGS?

Children are natural mimics—they act like their parents in spite of every attempt to teach them good manners.
ANONYMOUS

DAY **84**	**DATE:**
	182 days to go

The arms have almost reached their final proportions and length, but the legs are still quite short. The baby's muscle responses have been changed from mechanical and puppetlike to smooth and fluid, like a newborn's. The baby is 3⅓ inches long (87 mm) and weighs 1–2 ounces (43–60 g). (Remember that at the end of the second month, the baby measured about 1 inch (27 mm) in length and weighed about .04 ounce (1 g). Now, it is 3 times as long and more than 50 times as heavy!)

This day marks the end of the third full month of pregnancy—one full trimester, one third of the baby's total gestational time. Each day that you read, reflect, think, and learn about your pregnancy and your unborn child, you come closer to understanding your developing baby and to assimilating into the role of new (or renewed) parent.

Food Facts Magnesium barely qualifies as a major mineral because only about 1¾ ounces (50g) of magnesium can be found in the body of a 130-pound person, most of it in the bones. Pregnant women are advised to intake 450 mg of magnesium daily. Good food sources include nuts, legumes, cereal grains, dark-green vegetables, seafoods, chocolate, and cocoa.

Did You Know? The accuracy of your projected due date can be confirmed by examining the size of your uterus during prenatal visits. If there seems to be a large difference between the actual size and the expected size of the uterus, an ultrasound picture will be used to measure your baby.

notes

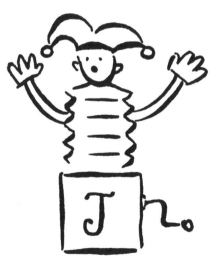

Children and chickens would ever be eating.

THOMAS TUSSER

Lunar Month 4

THINGS TO DO THIS MONTH:

Eat, especially when you have an appetite, and try to make your meals low in fat, small, and frequent.

Continue to get plenty of rest, drink plenty of fluids, and exercise in moderation.

Get sufficient vitamin C in your daily diet, since vitamin C can't be stored.

Take steps to avoid constipation; urinate when you feel the need.

Take steps to minimize or prevent varicose veins and backache.

Avoid secondhand smoke and consider quitting, if you smoke.

Avoid or minimize stretch marks on the surface of your skin.

Change position slowly (especially getting up after lying down) to avoid feeling faint.

Avoid gaining excess weight.

Report any fever or illness to your practitioner.

week 13

DAY
85

DATE:

181 days to go

The baby's neck is now well defined. The head now rests on the neck instead of the shoulders.

During the next month, your baby will grow faster than it ever has or ever will. Because of the rapid pace of growth this month, your baby needs you to eat sufficient, well-balanced meals and snacks. Give the baby's system plenty to work with by maintaining your well-balanced diet and drinking plenty of fluids.

Did You Know? You should know that nothing your practitioner does affects whether the baby's belly button points in or out, or its cosmetic appearance. The strength of the baby's tissues at the umbilical site makes this determination.

Childbirth in Other Cultures The Canadian Eskimos believe that the spirit or life force enters a baby early in the pregnancy and that the mother can talk to it and teach it during that time.

digested by the baby's maturing digestive tract as it practices for the time when unprocessed food will enter its system).

Your body naturally works to reduce the risks associated with pregnancy by increasing blood volume, increasing red blood cell count, getting more oxygen to tissues, and improving blood-clotting ability.

Chart your waist size and weight here.

WAIST SIZE   WEIGHT

Did You Know? After birth, your baby's hair will grow at a rate of about ½ inch (13 mm) a month.

Childbirth in Other Cultures Mayan women who have given birth go to sleep with the newborn baby in their arms and will not be separated from it until they resume their normal activities after twenty days.

notes

....
....
....
....
....
....
....
....
....

DAY
86

DATE:

180 days to go

Over the next three days, the baby's scalp hair pattern will be determined. Your baby is now able to practice breathing, swallowing, and sucking movements in preparation for life outside the womb. Some amniotic fluid is swallowed (to be

If any of us had a child that we thought was as bad as we know we were, we would have cause to start to worry.

WILL ROGERS

DAY 87	DATE:
	179 days to go

The rapid and sustained growth experienced by the baby this month enables it to be more dexterous and agile than before. For example, your baby can now turn its head, open its mouth, and press its lips together. Not bad for somebody who only weighs 1 ounce (28 g).

During pregnancy, your organ systems receive additional blood, according to their increased workload. The blood flow to the uterus and kidneys is thus increased, while the blood flow to the liver and the brain remains the same.

IMPORTANT You'll want to continue with your program of regular exercise, but avoid cycling, skiing, rollerblading, horseback riding, skateboarding, and surfing, because even experienced athletes can fall. Even though the baby is well protected, you'll want to avoid jarring your uterus at all times.

Food Facts Eating nuts can increase the fiber and starch in your diet, but cocktail nuts may not be the best choice during pregnancy. They have been fried in grease and oil and then are heavily salted. Try roasted, unsalted nuts.

notes

DAY 88	DATE:
	178 days to go

By today, the baby's scalp hair pattern has been determined.

You should feel less breast tenderness and tingling this month. Women generally feel more comfortable during the second trimester (Months 4, 5, and 6).

Food Facts Nuts packed in see-through containers can be checked for quality, but are subject to light degradation. The best are vacuum-packed nuts, since they are protected against light and air. Nuts like walnuts, cashews, almonds, and peanuts can be a significant source of protein during pregnancy (24–37 g a cup), but they are also a significant source of fat (64–77 g a cup).

Childbirth Then and Now Since the eighteenth century, Western women have been advised by their physicians to restrict their food intake during pregnancy in order to keep from gaining too much weight. At that time, malnutrition was prevalent, and malnourished girls often developed narrow, misshapen pelvises. Since such a pelvis made it difficult if not impossible to deliver a normal-sized baby and threatened the life of both the mother and the child, all women (even well-nourished ones) were encouraged to limit protein, calorie, salt, and carbohydrate intake during pregnancy. We know now that women without structural problems caused by deficiency diseases should not limit their nutrient or calorie intake during pregnancy, but such advice was widespread in the United States even as late as the 1960s.

Parenthood: The state of being better chaperoned than you were before marriage.
MARCELENE COX

DAY 89	DATE:
	177 days to go

The baby now has considerable hand and arm movement: it can make a fist, move its thumbs, and bend its wrists. It is also better able to grasp objects. All the body movements that the baby engages in right now constitute practice. It takes some time for the nervous system and the muscles to make smooth, synchronous movements. So these motions test the hook-ups within the neuromuscular system. The baby also is exercising its tiny muscles by moving them.

By now you may be experiencing some mild swelling or edema. It will be most noticeable in your ankles and feet, because of the effect of gravity on your tissues.

Swelling is an important symptom to report to your practitioner during your checkup. You might want to note when and where swelling occurs so you don't forget.

For Your Comfort
Elevate your feet when you sit and avoid standing for prolonged periods of time.

Childbirth in Other Cultures In the villages in Jordan in the Middle East, inhabitants advise that people be as careful of the child within its mother's womb as they are of the chicken in the egg.

DAY 90	DATE:
	176 days to go

The baby's heart pumps about 25 quarts of blood a day during the fourth month; that rate will increase to 300 quarts of blood a day by the time it is born.

By the end of this month, your growing uterus will rise out of the confines of your hipbones. Even though the baby is moving quite a bit, you still can't feel the movements because the baby doesn't bump into the walls of your uterus and doesn't have much muscle strength. You'll first notice the baby's movements in another seven weeks or so. It's ironic that while most mothers really want to feel their baby move and are so pleased when they finally do, those same movements will eventually keep them up at night and bump so hard they'd think the baby was wearing boots.

Childbirth in Other Cultures The Bambura of Africa and other African tribal groups believe that the spirit of the father's clan enters the baby early in pregnancy and the spirit of the mother's clan enters the baby at the naming ceremony, which takes place several months after birth.

Food Facts Lemons, like all citrus, are an excellent source of vitamin C during pregnancy. To get more juice from your lemon, bring it to room temperature or roll it before cutting.

$$1 + 1 = 2$$

Ask your child what he wants for dinner only if he's buying.
FRAN LEBOWITZ

DAY **9 1**	DATE: *175 days to go*

At this point in development, the baby has a considerable range of foot and leg movements: it can kick, turn its feet outward and inward, curl its toes, and fan its toes.

In another three or four weeks, tiny stretch marks (called striae gravidarum) may appear on your lower abdomen, buttocks, thighs, and breasts due to the rapid stretching of the skin. Stretch marks usually appear reddish or bluish at first; later they will fade to a silvery white.

Food Facts If cantaloupe or watermelon are available while you are pregnant, eat them, as they are excellent sources of vitamins A and C. Half of a 5-inch-diameter cantaloupe provides 6,540 IU of vitamin A (only 5,000 IU of vitamin A is required daily!). One-sixteenth of a two-pound watermelon provides 2,510 IU of vitamin A.

Did You Know? The hardest substance in your baby's body is tooth enamel.

How are you feeling today?

MOOD:

ENERGY:

APPETITE:

MORNING SICKNESS?

CRAVINGS?

notes

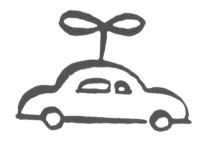

Of all animals, the boy is the most unmanageable.
PLATO

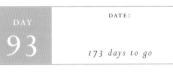

week 14

<table>
<tr><td>DAY
92</td><td>DATE:

174 days to go</td></tr>
</table>

<table>
<tr><td>DAY
93</td><td>DATE:

173 days to go</td></tr>
</table>

Rapid and sustained growth continues all this week. Over the next two days, the baby's head and neck will straighten as more bone is formed and the back muscles become stronger.

You may experience occasional nosebleeds and nasal stuffiness due to increases in blood volume and the effects of the hormone estrogen, which causes your nasal membranes to swell.

Did You Know? If you do experience a nosebleed, applying pressure to the sides of the nose (about halfway down, past the bony tissue) probably works best to stop the bleeding. Tip your head slightly back.

Childbirth Then and Now In England in the 1600s, pregnant women were expected to have unusual desires and cravings. The prevailing belief was that if a woman's desires were frustrated, their resulting anger could result in miscarriage. Thus, to prevent such problems, husbands were told by doctors to dote on their spouses.

The baby's head and neck have assumed more of a straight-line relationship.

Chances are you'll notice more weight gain during the next three months. It stands to reason that if your baby is growing rapidly, you should note some weight increases, too.

For Your Health Remember to limit unnecessary or excess weight gain. Extra weight will just be that much more difficult to lose after the baby is born.

Childbirth Then and Now In 1680, Johanna St. John in *Her Booke* suggested that the expectant woman take a dried toad and hang it around her waist to safeguard the pregnancy.

notes

....

....

....

....

....

....

....

....

....

....

All children wear the sign: "I want to be important NOW."
Many of our juvenile delinquency problems arise because nobody reads the sign.
DAN PURSUIT

DAY **94**	DATE:
	172 days to go

During this month, the baby's body will begin to grow faster than its head.

You may notice that some clear fluid can be expressed from your breasts—this is not colostrum (a yellowish fluid rich in protein and anti-bodies), which won't appear until the end of Week 16. It is fluid that has accumulated in your mammary glands due to the changing levels of hormones in your system.

Food Facts The best food sources of vitamin A are yellow vegetables and dried apricots. One cup of canned sweet potatoes offers 17,000 IU of vitamin A (5,000 is the daily requirement during pregnancy), one cup of pumpkin provides 14,590 IU, and one cup of dried apricots yields 16,350 IU. While vitamin A can be toxic in high doses (more than 5-10 times the recommended intake), the safest and easiest way to meet the body's vitamin A needs is through foods, not dietary supplements.

Childbirth in Other Cultures Historically, Native American women and their newborns plunged into a stream immediately after delivery. If no running water was available, the child was dipped in cold water as soon as it was born. Saltwater baths and washes were used by people who lived by the sea. The cold-water bath was considered to be an initiation of the newborn child into the troubles of this world.

DAY **95**	DATE:
	171 days to go

Over the next three days, the baby's toenails will begin to grow from their nail beds.

Nasal congestion is common during pregnancy as the mucous membranes swell. You may feel particularly congested during the winter months, when dry heated air circulates to warm the house, or if you have a cold; you also may be uncomfortable when it's warmer and allergies compound nasal stuffiness. Your ears may also feel full or stuffy.

If the full sensation in your nose or ears is accompanied by pain, fever, or flulike symptoms, check with your practitioner to make sure you don't have an infection.

Food Facts Consider eating seed vegetables like beans and peas during your pregnancy. They are among the best vegetable sources of iron and protein.

notes

....

....

....

....

....

....

....

....

....

In youth we learn, in age we understand.

MARIE VON EBNER-ESCHENBACH

DAY 96	DATE:
	170 days to go

The principles of exchange that govern the baby's blood supply make it impossible for the baby to completely deplete the mother's blood supply of nutrients, so there's always something left over for your system.

As the ligaments that support your uterus stretch, you may experience some abdominal pain.

Did You Know? You may be more comfortable sitting rather than standing. A heating pad might warm the abdominal and lower back muscles enough to relax them and provide some relief.

Food Facts Tannin is a bitter-tasting acid in coffee that increases as the coffee brews. To avoid excess tannin in your coffee: (1) never boil your coffee, (2) maintain the least amount of contact between the coffee and the boiling water (the drip method is best), (3) remove the coffee grounds as soon as the coffee is perked. Remember to limit your coffee intake during pregnancy to less than two cups per day.

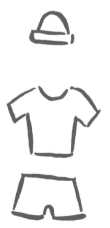

notes

DAY 97	DATE:
	169 days to go

The baby's head now appears upright, rather than curving down on the chest. The toenails are growing from their nail beds.

As your uterus shifts and relieves pressure from your bladder, you may find you don't have to urinate quite as frequently. Enjoy it while it lasts. Toward the end of your pregnancy, frequent urination will return. You might want to carry tissue and toilet seat covers with you in your purse, pack, or car in case you need to stop at facilities that are less than sanitary. Also, continue to take steps to avoid constipation.

Food Facts For your safety and the safety of your baby, eat organic fruit or fruits with peels that can be removed (like bananas, melons, and pineapples) so you don't unknowingly ingest herbicides and pesticides used when the fruit was grown.

Childbirth in Other Cultures The Luzon of the Philippines believe that if an expectant mother quarrels with her own mother or with her mother-in-law, she will have a difficult delivery.

The hardest job kids face today is learning good manners without seeing any.
FRED ASTAIRE

notes

DAY 98	DATE:
	168 days to go

The baby measures 4¾ inches long (120 mm) crown to rump and weighs 3¾ ounces (104.5 g), having more than doubled its dimensions in a mere two weeks.

You may notice that your veins are becoming more apparent because of the extra volume of blood created by your system to support the pregnancy. The average amount of blood lost during a completely normal birth is about one pint, or the amount that is given when donating one unit of blood.

For Your Comfort

If your veins are beginning to bulge, you'll want to guard against the pain and discomfort that can accompany varicose veins. Wear support stockings, gain no excess weight, elevate your feet when you can, move your ankles while sitting, and exercise to improve blood flow.

Food Facts Lettuce should be washed well before it is eaten, but it should never be soaked in water, since soaking extracts the vitamins. Even though lettuce is mostly water, it offers a fair amount of vitamin A value to your diet.

How are you feeling today?

Mood:

Energy:

Appetite:

Morning sickness?

Cravings?

Babies are such a nice way to start people.
Don Herold

week 15

DAY 99	DATE:
	167 days to go

DAY 100	DATE:
	166 days to go

During this entire week, the baby grows rapidly, with growth setting the stage for development later this month. The baby's weight will increase six times during this fourth month of pregnancy. Even then, the baby will only weigh 6 ounces (168 g), not even half a pound.

You probably still feel tired and sometimes out of energy. That's normal. Plenty of rest, good nutrition, and exercise should make you feel better.

Chart your waist size and weight here.

WAIST SIZE   WEIGHT

Childbirth Then and Now To hurry her labor, the Klamath Indian mother would tell her baby that a rattlesnake was coming to bite it, if it did not hurry out of the womb!

Food Facts When fruits are dried, about 50% of the water is removed. Dried fruits are a rich source of natural sugar plus all the vitamins and minerals contained in the fruit when it is fresh. Dried fruits are the ideal substitute for candy and are easy to carry with you.

Blood travels with considerable force through the umbilical cord, giving the cord the same kind of tension as a water-filled hose. The cord resists knotting and tends to straighten itself out as the baby moves about.

Change position slowly, especially if you are getting up from lying down, to avoid feeling faint or dizzy. During pregnancy, blood pressure changes that equalize pressure from changing positions occur more slowly.

IMPORTANT If you're feeling lightheaded, sit down and lower your head, or lie down and elevate your feet. Wait for the symptoms to pass before you attempt to stand.

Did You Know? The baby's link to the placenta is the umbilical cord. The placenta and umbilical cord develop only in animals that do not hatch from eggs. In other words, chickens don't have belly buttons.

notes

Children need love, especially when they do not deserve it.
HAROLD S. HULBERT

DAY	DATE:
101	*165 days to go*

With the help of the placenta and the umbilical cord, the baby's system is operating as it will after it's born. The baby has its own circulation, pumped by the heart, which at this developmental stage, pumps the equivalent of 25 quarts of blood (27.5 liters) a day.

The chances are good that you've noticed an increase in your appetite. Eating nutritious food provides fuel to sustain the baby's growth and to give you the energy you need to manage the "non-pregnant" aspects of your life.

Childbirth Then and Now Rural birth attendants in pioneer America were often neighbors and grannies. Their advice following childbirth, "Eat anything y'want except kraut and pickled beans, and stay in th'bed for ten days."

Food Facts Sardines are an excellent source of dietary calcium. Three ounces of sardines (drained) offer 372 mg of calcium, over a quarter of the pregnant woman's daily requirement (1,200 mg).

your baby is practicing all three of these reflex behaviors: sucking, swallowing, and blinking. It is also working on incorporating some additional reflexes, so that by the time it is born, the average full term baby will display more than seventy different reflex behaviors.

During this month, the placenta will become the main source of hormones needed to sustain the pregnancy and to prepare for the production of milk. Later, the placenta will play an important role in determining the changing hormone balance that will help to initiate labor and birth.

Childbirth in Other Cultures To the Jarara of South America, childbirth is such a normal event that it takes place in a location in full view of everyone.

Food Facts You can help safeguard your health and the environment by cutting down on fried foods. But if you must fry, season your pan before frying (wipe with an oiled paper towel) so you can avoid using environmentally hazardous sprays designed to keep foods from sticking.

notes

DAY	DATE:
102	*164 days to go*

The baby is getting bigger this week. It is also adding to its list of reflex behaviors. Reflexes are the automatic, unlearned behaviors a baby is born with. Most reflexes have survival value for the infant: blinking helps keep foreign objects out of their eyes and keeps their eyes moist; sucking and swallowing provide for the ingestion of nutrients. Right now,

Every beetle is a gazelle in the eyes of its mother.
Moorish proverb

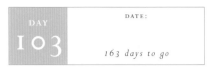

DATE:

DAY 103

163 days to go

During this month, the baby grows so much that it reaches half the length it will attain by birth.

During the next couple of weeks (Weeks 16 to 18, generally), your baby's growth might be assessed by either amniocentesis or an AFP (alphafetoprotein) screening test, both of which also screen for birth defects. The AFP is a test of the mother's blood; an amniocentesis involves insertion of a needle through the abdomen and uterine wall to remove some amniotic fluid, which is then tested.

For Your Information AFP is a substance manufactured during pregnancy and is in detectable levels in the mother's blood-stream. The first step in AFP screening involves testing your blood to see if those levels are considered to be high. High levels of AFP can be an indication of Down's syndrome or that your baby's brain and/or spinal cord might not be developing properly (this is rare, affecting only 2-4% of all pregnancies). If AFP levels are high, follow-up testing by amniocentesis would be recommended. Amniotic fluid cells would be examined for signs of metabolic and/or genetic and chromosomal problems. Amniocentesis is useful in the diagnosis of Down's syndrome, some metabolic and genetic disorders, and in testing the maturity of the baby's lungs. Should you be a candidate for AFP screening or amniocentesis, be sure to ask questions of your practitioner so you can be clear about the risks and benefits for you and your baby.

Food Facts Bell peppers are a great source of vitamin C. Since one raw pepper provides 94 mg of vitamin C (the daily requirement during pregnancy is 80–100 mg), consider adding some to your salad on a regular basis. A cooked bell pepper provides 70 mg of vitamin C and it is good in soups, bean dishes, omelettes, meat dishes, and stir-fry.

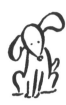

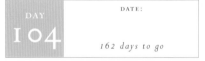

DAY 104

DATE:

162 days to go

During this month, the baby and the placenta are nearly equal in size, but the baby will soon grow larger than the placenta.

As your baby grows larger and stronger, it becomes more and more likely that you'll actually begin to feel it move. At first the baby feels like a butterfly fluttering in your abdomen. The very earliest movements are reported around this time during the pregnancy (Weeks 14 or 15). More likely, you will feel your baby move at the same time as the majority of women do: sometime around Week 18, 19, or 20.

Did You Know? Worldwide, 80% of newborns are delivered by midwives. The word midwife comes from Old English words meaning "with the woman" (*mid* = with and *wif* = woman). Similarly, in Latin the midwife is the *cum-mater* and in Portuguese and Spanish, she is the *comadrona.* Among the ancient Jews, she is the "wise woman," a characterization reflected both in the modern German term *weise frau,* and in the modern French, *sage-femme.*

Never allow your child to call you by your first name. He hasn't known you long enough.
FRAN LEBOWITZ

Food Facts Vitamin A plays a role in maintaining the health of the mucous membranes and skin and promotes bone growth. Tomato juice is an excellent source of vitamin A. One-half cup of tomato juice offers 970 IU of vitamin A, about 20% of your day's requirement during pregnancy.

DAY	DATE:
105	*161 days to go*

This was a week of rapid, whole-body growth for your baby. Existing structures became larger and more well-developed, but no new structures were formed.

The chances are good that this week's growth spurt for your baby also resulted in a growth spurt for you.

Food Facts Potatoes are an inexpensive, nutritious food during pregnancy. Baked or boiled potatoes with skins left on offer 80–90 calories, 3 g of protein, essentially no fat, and 1.4–1.7 mg of niacin. Mashed potatoes (made with milk and butter) offer 4 g of protein in a one cup serving, 330 IU of vitamin A, 185 calories, and 8 g of fat. Ten baked, two-inch french fries or ten 2-inch-diameter potato chips contain about 120 calories and 5 and 8 g of fat, respectively.

Childbirth in Other Cultures If a baby girl is born to a Mayan woman living in the Yucatán peninsula, the mother will have the baby's ears pierced before she is sixty minutes old. Mayans believe that babies don't feel anything so soon after birth; a day later, she would be "paying attention."

notes

How are you feeling today?

MOOD:

ENERGY:

APPETITE:

MORNING SICKNESS?

CRAVINGS?

Level with your child by being honest. Nobody spots a phony quicker than a child.
MARY MacCRACKEN

week 16

DAY
106

DATE:

160 days to go

Over the next three days, pads will begin to form on the baby's fingertips and toes.

A thin, whitish vaginal discharge called leukorrhea is normally secreted during pregnancy. You may notice this secretion becoming heavier as your pregnancy continues.

Contact your practitioner if the vaginal discharge changes color (becomes yellowish or greenish), thickens, or is accompanied by burning, itching, or pain during urination. These may be symptoms that require attention.

Food Facts Both the baby and the placenta need iron, since iron supports the dramatic increase in blood volume and red blood cell production. Prune juice has ten to forty times more iron than other fruit juices.

DAY
107

DATE:

159 days to go

By today, meconium (the early fecal waste material) will begin to accumulate in the baby's bowel. This material is the product of cell loss, digestive secretions, and swallowed amniotic fluid and is the result of the digestive system practicing digestion while the baby is still in the womb.

Your carbohydrate needs will increase during these last two trimesters of pregnancy. Carbohydrates provide your body with energy and can be found in sugars, starches, and fiber.

Food Facts Low-fat, high-carbohydrate fruits and vegetables include canned peas, potatoes, sweet potatoes, red kidney beans, lima beans, blackeyed peas, split peas, green beans, canned corn, catsup, sweetened applesauce, dried apricots, bananas, canned cherries, pitted dates, canned fruit cocktail, canned or dried peaches, canned pineapple, canned pears, cooked prunes, raisins, frozen strawberries, and watermelon. The reason that canned vegetables and fruits are higher in carbohydrates than fresh vegetables and fruits is that the canning process adds refined sugar to the natural sugars already found in these foods.

Childbirth Then and Now During the nineteenth century in North America, most births were attended by midwives, relatives, or friends. Physicians were typically mistrusted and consulted only in the most desperate cases. For Native Americans, older women of the tribes were assumed to be especially knowledgeable regarding childbirth.

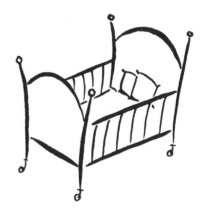

The real message in dealing with a five-year-old is that in no time at all,
you will begin to sound like a five-year-old.

JEAN KERR

DAY	DATE:
108	*158 days to go*

By today, the baby has pads on its fingertips and toes that will develop the characteristic swirls and creases of the finger and toe prints.

As you identify yourself more and more with being pregnant, you might find that even if you're excited about having a baby, you sometimes feel scared, worried, and ambivalent about the future. You should know that pregnancy is a mix of both positive and negative feelings and that your particular feelings are perfectly normal. While worry cannot help by itself, being worried about the future might help you plan and solve problems now so that some of the burden of adjusting to a new baby is lessened. Don't worry if you don't have all the answers—no one does. The good thing is that you've got questions and you can find answers if you just ask. Physicians, midwives, friends, parents, and counselors are all good resources.

IMPORTANT Remember: the only stupid question is the one that doesn't get asked.

Food Facts If you need a quick pick-me-up beverage, try these high-carbohydrate, low-fat choices: apricot juice, grape juice, lemonade, limeade, orange juice, grapefruit juice, and cranberry juice cocktail.

DAY	DATE:
109	*157 days to go*

The baby's eyes now look forward rather than to the sides.

While the placenta serves to keep the baby healthy, it also plays a role in safeguarding your health. The placenta can synthesize globulins, natural ingredients in the blood that prevent infection. While most of the globulins are dispensed to the baby, you receive some as well, especially during the last three months of pregnancy.

Food Facts One cup of cooked oatmeal provides a significant amount of protein (5 g), 1.4 mg of iron, and half of the vitamin B_1 you require each day during pregnancy. Instant hot cereals are not as nutritious, but you don't need them—in only five more minutes, you can cook a hot cereal that retains much more of its nutrient value.

Childbirth Then and Now In colonial America, it was common to have the laboring woman seated on her husband's lap, he being seated on a chair. He would hold onto the woman around the top of her abdomen or under her arms. As a male writer commented in 1882: "This position was certainly not a bad one for all parties with the exception of the husband who, in tedious cases, suffered rather severely; but then this little tax on his affectionate nature was, in those days, considered the very least return he could make for the mischief he had occasioned."

I have found that the best way to give advice to your children is to find out what they want and then to advise them to do it.

HARRY S. TRUMAN

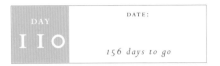

DAY 110
DATE:

156 days to go

Over the next two days, the ears will move to their final positions.

From this week on, your heart has to work 40–50% harder to support your pregnancy. Generally, this added workload doesn't pose a problem—a healthy heart can cope with the increased demand.

If you can't quit smoking, cut down, and if you can't cut down, talk to your practitioner about nicotine substitutes and habit management.

IMPORTANT Weigh the pros and cons of medications carefully; substitute sparkling juice drinks or flavored waters for alcohol; and if you smoke, remember that your baby is exposed to anything you're exposed to—consider quitting.

Did You Know? An average of 10,501 babies are born each day in the United States.

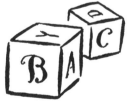

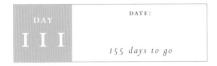

DAY 111
DATE:

155 days to go

Many of the baby's bones have begun to harden.

After you have a meal, the baby receives its nutrients within a hour or two.

Food Facts Consider seasoning your food with fresh seasonings like garlic, onion, ginger, chili pepper, and lemon instead of with salt. For some women, limiting salt intake can help reduce fluid retention and swelling during pregnancy. Check with your practitioner about salt in your diet.

Childbirth in Other Cultures There is considerable cultural variation about whether a pregnant woman should take food or fast during labor. Pawnee Indians of North America do not permit the woman to eat or drink after the first pain of labor. On the other hand, African Hottentots feed laboring women soup to keep them strong.

notes

....
....
....
....
....
....
....
....
....
....
....

Who takes the child by the hand takes the mother by the heart.
GERMAN PROVERB

	DATE:
DAY **112**	
	154 days to go

By this time, if your baby is a boy, the male prostate gland has developed. Also, the process of myelinization has begun. Myelinization involves coating the nerves with a fatty substance called myelin to speed nerve cell transmission and to insulate the nerves so messages are uninterrupted. The baby that has been growing so rapidly inside you now measures 5½ inches (140 mm) in length: big enough for you to cradle in the palm of your hand.

By now you may have felt your baby's fluttery movement for the first time. If not, this next month will have that in store for you. The baby has been moving steadily. If you haven't yet felt the movement, you most likely will during these next two weeks. Again, don't expect bumps and thumps right now. The feelings will be more like a growling stomach, a bubble bursting, butterflies in the stomach—even indigestion or hunger pains.

Food Facts Cheese is a good food choice during pregnancy because it is a concentrated source of many of the nutrients found in milk. The protein obtained from cheese is of equal quality to meat protein, and cheese usually costs much less.

Did You Know? One ounce of Cheddar or Swiss cheese provides 20% of the day's calcium requirements and 10% of the day's protein, along with 100 calories and 8–9 grams of fat.

notes

How are you feeling today?

Mood:

Energy:

Appetite:

Morning Sickness?

Cravings?

Feel the dignity of a child. Do not feel superior to him, for you are not.
Robert Henri

Lunar Month 5

Things to Do This Month:

Avoid strenuous work and follow the suggestions provided this month to prevent backache.

Sleep or rest on your left side; rest when you feel tired.

Wear comfortable, nonrestrictive clothing.

Avoid getting overheated; keep fresh air circulating and avoid fumes that might be toxic.

Report severe gum pain or discomfort to your dentist.

Prevent urinary tract infection.

Prevent iron deficiency anemia by including sufficient iron in your diet.

Keep your blood sugar level stable by eating frequently and carrying a snack with you.

Prevent leg and foot cramps and minimize swelling of your ankles, feet, and hands.

Prevent hemorrhoids by avoiding constipation.

week 17

DAY 113	DATE:
	153 days to go

DAY 114	DATE:
	152 days to go

The baby's external ears now stand out from its head. Over this next month, the baby will gain about 2 inches (51 mm) in height and nearly 26 ounces (728 g) in weight.

Congratulations, you've now been pregnant for four months! In two more weeks, you'll be halfway to your baby's birthdate.

Think About It Whether your pregnancy has gone quickly or slowly doesn't matter as much as whether it's going well. Remember—you are the architect of your baby's environment. Pampering yourself actually means pampering your baby: don't feel selfish if you need extra rest time, choose to cut down on activities, or want another helping at mealtime.

Childbirth in Other Cultures While many cultures prescribe that only women can assist a laboring woman, the Lepcha of the Himalayas have no sex preference: any knowledgeable person can attend to the birth and help the mother.

notes

....

....

....

....

....

....

Over the next two days, lanugo (temporary downy hair) will begin to appear on the baby's head and body. No one knows what purpose lanugo serves, but by the time the baby is born, most of it will have disappeared.

You'll gain most of your weight in the next three months. Generally, you might expect an average increase of a pound a week until Month 7. Weight gain will be mostly uneven, though. It's much more common to gain nothing one week, 2 lbs. (896 g) the next, ½ pound (224 g) the following week, and so on. Take care not to get too tired, since the rapid growth of the baby this month will compound the burden on your heart, lungs, and kidneys.

Chart your waist size and weight here.

WAIST SIZE	WEIGHT

Food Facts Calcium builds your baby's bones and teeth. Even though fresh vegetables are generally poor sources of calcium compared to milk and milk products, dark green leafy vegetables do offer significant amounts.

For Your Information Four 1-cup servings of collard greens, dandelion greens, or turnip greens will satisfy your daily calcium requirements.

Children in families are like flowers in a bouquet:
there's always one determined to face in an opposite direction from the way the arranger desires.
MARCELENE COX

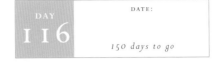

DAY 115	DATE: *151 days to go*

Last month the baby grew from 3½ inches (89 mm) long to 5½ inches (140 mm) long. That's a substantial size increase. This month you can expect the same dramatic growth. In four short weeks, the baby will grow from 5½ inches (140 mm) in length to 8–10 inches (203–254 mm) long!

As you gain more weight, you may want to switch to fuller, less restrictive clothing made from lighter-weight fabrics. This will keep you more comfortable as your body temperature increases.

Food Facts Corn is a good source of pregnancy-supporting vitamins. Since the sugar in the kernels begins to turn to starch after harvesting, fresh corn is best eaten immediately after purchase. Do not remove the husks until just before cooking. Three minutes in boiling water sets the milk in the corn that is rich in flavor and nutrients. Do not salt the water, as this tends to harden the kernels.

Childbirth in Other Cultures Most West African tribal cultures believe that a baby is so close to the spirit world that both the baby and mother are vulnerable to the influence of evil spirits. For protection, the mother is told to wear special amulets and charms and to avoid doing anything that would attract the attention of the spirits.

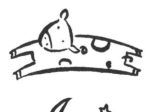

DAY 116	DATE: *150 days to go*

If your baby is a girl, primitive egg cells are now within the ovaries. Baby girls are born with all the eggs they will ever have in their ovaries. By the time she is ready to have a family of her own, your daughter's eggs will be as old as she is.

You may notice that your back begins to ache as your pregnancy continues. Most pregnancy backaches consist of low back pain, because the narrowest part of your back (your waist) has to balance your growing uterus and because the normally stable joints in your pelvis begin to loosen somewhat to make childbirth easier. Since backache is so common during pregnancy, over the next week or so we'll list ten suggestions, one at a time, for avoiding or minimizing backache:

NO MORE ACHING BACK *Suggestion #1:* Maintain good posture. Pretend there is a string running through your backbone and out the top of your head. Imagine being pulled up by the string. Align your head, neck, backbone, and pelvis. Feel yourself lift and straighten. Consciously straighten your alignment when you feel yourself slouch. Also, avoid tilting your pelvis forward.

Childbirth in Other Cultures Hopi women of the American Southwest are encouraged to get up early every morning and not to sit around during pregnancy. The Sanpoil tribe goes even further. For their pregnant woman, a regular program of exercise, mainly walking and swimming, is prescribed.

For there is no kind that had any other first beginning. For all men have one entrance into life.
THE WISDOM OF SOLOMON IN THE APOCRYPHA

DAY 117	DATE:
	149 days to go

Over the next two days, the vernix caseosa begins to form. This is a creamy-looking substance that covers the baby's skin in order to protect it and its developing glands and sensory cells. The vernix is composed of dead skin, oil from the oil-bearing glands of the baby's skin, and the lanugo.

By this time you may have noticed the appearance of a mottled area of pigmentation that extends beyond the existing areola and sometimes covers half of the breast. Called the secondary areola, this pigmentation change in breast tissue is temporary, but may last for as long as twelve months after the birth before it disappears.

No MORE ACHING BACK *Suggestion #2:* Avoid extra weight gain. The more extra weight you put on, the more weight your back will have to balance. If you cut out all the junk food and food with high fat content, any weight you gain will be "healthy weight."

Childbirth in Other Cultures A custom among the nineteenth century Loango of Africa was that as long as the umbilical stump was still on the child, no male being, not even the father, would be admitted into the presence of the newborn for fear that the child would fall into evil ways.

notes

Children are remarkable for their intelligence and ardor, for their curiosity, their intolerance of shams, the clarity and ruthlessness of their vision.

ALDOUS HUXLEY

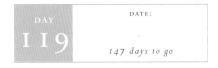

DAY	DATE:
118	148 days to go

The vernix has begun to form over the baby's body.

In addition to breast changes, blotchy areas of pigmentation may also appear on your forehead and on the sides of your face. This pigmentation is called the "mask of pregnancy" (chloasma) and usually fades and disappears after birth. Because exposure to the sun can further darken the area and make it less likely to fade, a sunscreen is recommended. The pigmentation will fade within a few months after childbirth.

NO MORE ACHING BACK *Suggestion #3:* When you sit, elevate your legs or use an ergonomically designed chair to take the pressure off your back.

Childbirth Then and Now "Two or three years ago (1879/1880), an Indian party of Flat Heads and Kootenais men, women, and children, set out for a hunting trip. On a severely cold winter's day, one of the women, allowing the party to proceed, dismounted from her horse, spread an old buffalo robe upon the snow and gave birth to a child which was immediately followed by the placenta. Having attended to everything as well as the circumstances permitted, she wrapped up the young one in a blanket, mounted her horse, and overtook the party before they had noticed her absence." (Engelmann, *Labor Among Primitive Peoples,* 1882)

DAY	DATE:
119	147 days to go

From now until the baby is born, the placenta will grow in diameter but not in thickness. It will grow to over 6 inches (152 mm) in diameter.

Occasionally, the baby will hiccup, causing a rhythmic jarring of your abdomen every two to four seconds or so. While there is no air to intake, hiccuping in the womb involves the same sort of muscular reactions as in an air-breathing child. The hiccuping generally stops in about a half hour. By the time you go to bed tonight, you will have been pregnant for eighteen weeks.

Food Facts While meats, cheeses, and eggs add saturated fats to your diet during pregnancy, the fat portion of nuts and seeds is highly unsaturated and is better for your heart and arteries. Coconuts are the exception—they're high in saturated fat and not a good source of protein. That's why it's good to look for products with no tropical oils.

Childbirth in Other Cultures Music is played throughout labor for the Navaho women of the American Southwest.

How are you feeling today?

MOOD: ....

ENERGY: ....

APPETITE: ....

MORNING SICKNESS? ....

CRAVINGS? ....

Children . . . they string our joys, like jewels bright, upon the thread of years.
EDWARD A. GUEST

week 18

DAY	DATE:
1 2 0	*146 days to go*

DAY	DATE:
1 2 1	*145 days to go*

By today, heat-producing brown fat has begun to form on the baby's neck, chest, and crotch areas. Brown fat has a protective function: it helps keep the baby warm in cold environments. Brown fat exists in newborns, but only vestiges of brown fat remain to adulthood.

The linea alba, or white line, between your navel and pubic hair line, generally becomes clearly pigmented during pregnancy. After it is pigmented, it is known as the linea nigra.

No More Aching Back *Suggestion #4:* Wear shoes that give your feet support. Some heel is actually better than no heel at all, but don't go over two inches—you might lose your balance and fall.

Food Facts Nuts are an excellent source of fiber during pregnancy, but watch out for added coloring and too much salt, even though the shells on nuts guard against nutritional depletion and chemical invasion. (Pistachios are the exception here. If the choice is between dyed nuts and the natural cream-colored ones, choose the latter.) Cashews are the only variety of nut never sold in the shell.

Over the next two days, the baby's eyebrows will begin to form.

If you are a brunette, your pigmentation changes will be more pronounced than if you have naturally lighter hair. Your pituitary gland seems to be responsible for the pigmentation changes: it releases more melanin (pigmentation)-stimulating hormone during pregnancy than when you're not pregnant.

No More Aching Back *Suggestion #5:* If you have to lift something, first make sure it's not too heavy, then lift with your legs—not with your back. Bend at your knees, keeping your back fairly straight, grasp the object, then straighten your legs to lift. If you can get into the habit of lifting with your legs, you'll protect yourself from back injury and strain even when you aren't pregnant.

Food Facts Since you are advised to limit caffeine and coffee intake during pregnancy, you will want to have the tastiest coffee you can when you treat yourself to an occasional cup. Store your ground coffee in the refrigerator in an airtight container to preserve its freshness and flavor. The essential flavoring in coffee comes from caffeol, a substance that is lost by exposure to air. In order for caffeol to be released, the beans must be ground. So for maximum flavor, freshly ground beans are best.

Raising a child is like reading a very long mystery story;
you have to wait for a generation to see how it turns out.
ANONYMOUS

DAY	DATE:
122	*144 days to go*

The baby sleeps and wakes as much as a newborn does now. When the baby sleeps, it characteristically settles into its favorite position or "lie." Some babies always sleep with their chins resting on the chest, while others tilt their heads back.

NO MORE ACHING BACK *Suggestion #6:* Try to avoid carrying objects in your arms. Weight in your arms only adds to the weight already out in front of you. Carry objects down at your sides, use a luggage carrier or other similar tote device with wheels, or ask for help.

Childbirth Then and Now The custom among the West Micronesians on the Isle of Jap during the nineteenth century was to begin to dilate a pregnant woman's cervix at least one month before delivery was expected. The leaves of a certain plant were rolled into a tight tube and inserted into the cervix. When dilated to that size, a thicker roll was introduced. This prelabor dilation of the cervix made labor faster and less painful, but the procedure itself caused some cramping and discomfort.

DAY	DATE:
123	*143 days to go*

Over the next three days, fine scalp hair will start to form on the baby's head. (This is the permanent hair, not lanugo.) Even this "permanent hair" will begin to fall out in the second week following birth, to be replaced gradually by coarser, thicker hair.

NO MORE ACHING BACK *Suggestion #7:* Ask your practitioner about exercises to strengthen and maintain your back muscles.

Childbirth Then and Now The obstetric chair—a chair with a back and false bottom—was first developed for use in Europe in the 1540s. Today, chairs are used by some physicians in some hospitals and birth centers.

Food Facts As beneficial as protein is now that you're pregnant, too much protein could be as harmful as too little. Stay within the recommended dietary guidelines and consult with your practitioner about adjustments.

notes

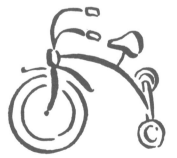

A happy childhood can't be cured. Mine'll hang around my neck like a rainbow.
HORTENSE CALISHER

DAY	DATE:
124	*142 days to go*

In the next three days, the vernix caseosa becomes noticeable on the baby's skin.

N O M O R E A C H I N G B A C K *Suggestion #8:* Remember to sit with your legs elevated or with your legs bent and your feet supported on a footstool.

Did You Know? From Week 12 to Week 20, the placenta weighs as much as, if not more than the baby, because it must deal with the metabolic processes of nutrition. The fetal organs are not yet sufficiently mature to process food.

Food Facts It's wise to limit fat intake to not more than 30% of your total calories for the day.

notes

DAY	DATE:
125	*141 days to go*

By today, hair will have begun to form on the baby's head. In another month, the head hair may be up to an inch long.

N O M O R E A C H I N G B A C K *Suggestion #9:* Avoid standing for prolonged periods of time. If you must stand for a while, stand with one foot elevated on a footstool.

Food Facts High-fat foods include butter, margarine, and oil, but don't forget to include bacon, olives, and avocados. When you eat bacon, you are not eating a protein food, you are eating a fat food. Avocados contribute essentially pure fat to your pregnancy diet: one-eighth of an avocado has as much fat as one slice of bacon or one pat of butter.

Childbirth Then and Now In the 1800s, inhabitants of the island of Ceram, north of Australia, tied laboring women to a post or tree with their hands above their heads. Often, the woman was semisuspended. This practice seemed to cut labor time—so that women could return to their responsibilities sooner.

The best way to keep children home is to make the home atmosphere pleasant—and let the air out of the tires.
DOROTHY PARKER

| DAY **126** | DATE:

140 days to go |

By this time, if your baby is a girl, the uterus has completely formed. As Week 18 ends, the baby weighs about 11 ounces (308 g) and measures about 6⅓ inches (160 mm) in length.

The baby's movements are becoming stronger as the ossification process continues and soft cartilage is hardened into bone. Mothers who are slim may feel their babies move much earlier than heavier moms will.

For Your Information The baby's umbilical stump is usually about an inch long. Sometimes it is painted with a purple dye to reduce the chance of infection. The cord is usually shriveled at the end of the first week, and the stump usually falls off between seven and eighteen days later.

Childbirth in Other Cultures Those attending the birth will often talk to the laboring woman to help her relax, to encourage her, and to reassure her. Mayan birth attendants cheer the mother on with a repetitive chant if she seems to be tiring.

How are you feeling today?

Mood:

Energy:

Appetite:

Baby Movement?

Contractions?

notes

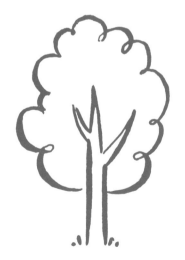

You can learn many things from children. How much patience you have, for instance.

Franklin P. Jones

week 19

DAY	DATE:
127	*139 days to go*

 Over the next three days, the baby's legs will approach their final relative proportions.

NO MORE ACHING BACK *Suggestion #10:* Sleep on a firm mattress that offers good back support. If your mattress is sagging, you can shore it up somewhat by putting a piece of plywood under it. You may also find that sleeping on the floor makes your back feel great (it's just difficult to know how to situate your bulging tummy).

If your back continues to bother you, avoid medication and call your practitioner.

Childbirth in Other Cultures Among the Dayak people of Borneo, a medicine man and his assistant visit a woman having a difficult labor. The assistant would stand outside the hut with a moon-colored stone tied to his belly. The medicine man, massaging and soothing the woman, would shout instructions to him to move the stone in imitation of the baby's movements, an act of magical transference.

Chart your waist size and weight here.

WAIST SIZE   WEIGHT

DAY	DATE:
128	*138 days to go*

The amniotic fluid is the perfect substance to support the baby's movement. The baby can move in any way its brain and muscles direct: spinning, jackknifing, turning, and somersaulting. The amniotic fluid keeps them buoyant, warm, and clean. It even gives them something to occasionally swallow so they can practice digesting and excreting waste.

The amniotic fluid that surrounds your baby is completely replaced by your system every three to four hours. Drinking plenty of fluids helps support that replacement and keeps your tissues functioning well, too.

Food Facts Juices are excellent beverages during pregnancy. Technically speaking, a "juice drink" is 50% juice, an "ade" is 25% juice, and a "fruit drink" is only 10% juice.

For Your Health Fluids are essential for good health and efficient functioning during pregnancy, since water makes up 55–60% of your body's weight. Drinking six to eight 8-ounce glasses of water or juice daily is recommended during pregnancy.

Before I got married, I had six theories about bringing up children; now I have six children and no theories.
JOHN WILMOT, EARL OF ROCHESTER

DAY 129

DATE:

137 days to go

Your baby's legs have now approached their final relative proportions. You'll notice that when the baby is born, its arms and legs appear rather short. That's normal. They'll get longer when the child moves from crawling to walking.

Sleeping position becomes an important consideration during pregnancy. You'll want to try to sleep on your side rather than on your back or your stomach.

Did You Know? If you can fall asleep on your left side—preferably with one leg crossed over the other and a pillow between them—you can maximize blood flow to the baby, reduce swelling in legs and feet, and improve the collection and elimination of waste. Sleeping exclusively on your back can actually interfere with blood flow back to your heart and increases backache. Sleeping on your stomach (on a conventional mattress) is usually just plain uncomfortable. If you wake up and notice you're on your stomach or your back, don't worry. Just roll over to your left side and try it again.

Food Facts Five small olives are the equivalent of 5 g of fat and have 45 calories.

notes

DAY 130

DATE:

136 days to go

In about a week, lanugo will completely cover the baby's body, although it will be concentrated around the head, neck, and face.

Your hair and nails tend to grow rapidly now that you're pregnant because of improved circulation and metabolism caused by pregnancy hormones. If you've ever wanted long, chip-resistant nails, now's the time.

If you go to a salon to have your nails done, sit in a well-ventilated area. Sometimes the fumes from the polishes, acrylic preparations, and acetone products can be quite strong.

For Your Health You'll want to check with your practitioner about any other risks associated with the salon.

People who say they sleep like a baby usually don't have one.
LEO J. BURKE

DAY 131	DATE: 135 days to go

The baby's heart is growing stronger and stronger. By this time (after Week 18), your baby's heartbeat can be detected by a stethoscope. If they forget to offer, ask if you can listen during your next prenatal visit.

You may notice that your gums are sensitive and sometimes swell and bleed. Like other changes, gum sensitivity results from increased levels of pregnancy hormones.

Check with your dentist if you experience severe gum pain or discomfort.

Did You Know? The umbilical cord is so well engineered that the bloodstream travels at four miles an hour and completes the round-trip through the cord and through the baby in only thirty seconds.

DAY 132	DATE: 134 days to go

The baby's arms and legs move with noticeably more force now as the muscles strengthen and the bones become stronger. The baby's sleep habits begin to appear—periods of drowsiness and sleep alternate with periods of activity. Sometimes the mother can detect and anticipate these cycles.

You may notice that you're feeling a little more emotionally stable and are experiencing fewer mood swings. Some irritability and absent-mindedness or forgetfulness are common. After all, you're probably still tired much of the time and you may be distracted by thoughts of the baby.

Food Facts Peanut butter is a very rich source of protein during pregnancy. Theoretically, peanut butter should be nothing more than ground nuts. However, read labels carefully: commercial peanut butters with added salt, sugar, and oils can be up to 55% fat.

Childbirth in Other Cultures In the United States, most women lie prone when they give birth. However, in most other cultures, women give birth in vertical positions: kneeling, sitting, squatting, standing, even being suspended from ropes or poles. Being upright has the advantage of speeding labor by working with the force of gravity.

Nothing has a stronger influence psychologically on their environment,
and especially on their children, than the unlived lives of the parents.

CARL JUNG

DAY 133	DATE: *133 days to go*

Right now the baby looks like a miniature newborn. Its face looks peaceful with closed eyes, nostrils, and a nicely formed mouth. Every once in a while, its thumb or finger will slip into the mouth and the baby will practice sucking.

Break out the sparkling apple juice—today is an important milestone in your pregnancy! You're now at the halfway point: nineteen weeks accomplished, nineteen weeks to go. From now on, your body will be preparing to give birth and your baby will be preparing for life outside your uterus.

Did You Know? Twins can sometimes be identified by separate heart sounds, especially if their heartbeats differ in rate by more than ten beats a minute.

Food Facts Vitamins D, E, and K are called "fat-soluble" vitamins because they are stored in abundance in the adipose (or fatty) tissues of the body. Therefore, it takes a long period of deficiency for the body to be depleted of these vitamins, even during pregnancy.

How are you feeling today?

MOOD:

ENERGY:

APPETITE:

BABY MOVEMENT?

CONTRACTIONS?

notes

Too often we give children answers to remember rather than problems to solve.
ROGER LEWIN

week 20

DAY	DATE:
134	*132 days to go*

During this week, the baby's brain will begin to grow rapidly. This rapid growth will continue until the child is five years old.

The baby may be roused from sleep by external sounds or movements: sudden loud noises, loud music, even the vibrations of a car or washing machine can stir the baby into activity.

By this time in your pregnancy, your practitioner may recommend that you reduce your level of exertion at work or even change job duties if your work involves strenuous lifting, bending below your waist, carrying, or climbing ladders or stairs. The idea is to avoid physical stress and strain that could tax your pregnancy.

For Your Information "Spider veins" (bright red elevations of the skin radiating from a central body) may develop on your chest, neck, face, arms, and legs. Like other vein changes, these, too, tend to disappear after childbirth.

notes

DAY	DATE:
135	*131 days to go*

By today, the baby's eyebrows and head hair will be visible. No matter how dark its hair will become, the baby's hair is now completely unpigmented. The eyebrows look like white streaks, and the hair on the baby's head is also white and very short.

By this time in pregnancy, iron-deficiency anemia may develop. More than 90% of women may be slightly anemic before they become pregnant, and about 20% of women are treated for iron-deficiency anemia during their pregnancy. If you don't have sufficient iron in your diet, your body doesn't produce as many red blood cells, and fewer red blood cells means less circulating oxygen in your system. Women with anemia may feel weak, tired, and out of breath and may even faint.

Did You Know? Preventing iron-deficiency anemia is easy. The best food sources of iron include calf liver (avoid beef liver since it might contain the hormones used to speed the cow's growth), blackstrap molasses, roast beef, ground beef, lima beans, soybeans, prunes, and turkey. Your practitioner might also prescribe a daily iron supplement.

Childbirth in Other Cultures Umbilical cord cutting is an important ritual in many cultures. Among some tribal cultures in the Philippines, the cord is measured until it touches the baby's forehead and is then cut. The extra length of cord insures that the baby will be "wise."

We call a child's mind "small" simply by habit; perhaps it is larger than ours, for it can take in almost anything without effort.
CHRISTOPHER MORLEY

DAY 136	DATE:
	130 days to go

At this point, the baby is very lean. Only about 1% of its body weight is due to fat. This proportion will change in the next weeks and months, as the fat the baby accumulates becomes food reserves to draw on after birth.

While dizziness or fainting may be a sign of anemia, it may also indicate that your blood-sugar level is low. To keep your blood-sugar level stable, eat frequent, small meals and carry a snack with you for a quick blood-sugar level lift. Also, don't get overheated. Open a window if you need fresh air and wear layers of clothing so you can remove them as needed.

Did You Know? A blood test is used to diagnose iron-deficiency anemia. Fortunately, while pregnant women may suffer symptoms, unborn babies rarely do. The mother's iron supply is depleted to serve the pregnancy, and if there isn't sufficient dietary iron to rebuild her reserves, she suffers the consequences.

Childbirth in Other Cultures The Punjabi of India and the Yahgan of Tierra del Fuego massage a woman's back and abdomen during labor. Other cultures help her push by applying pressure to her abdomen, squeezing her during contractions, or wrapping her with a belt or a binder during labor.

DAY 137	DATE:
	129 days to go

Sometime during the next three days, lanugo covers the baby's body.

You may continue to notice leg and foot cramps and some mild swelling (edema) of the ankles and feet. Prolonged standing, fatigue, and too much phosphorus and too little calcium in your diet may be responsible for cramping. Make adjustments where necessary so you can be as comfortable as possible. The easiest way to reduce phosphorus intake is to cut down on the amount of animal protein ingested.

Food Facts In order to reduce the amount of saturated fat in your diet, oil can successfully replace butter in cooking. When you cook, use 1 cup (a scant cup) of oil for every cup of butter needed. Safflower oil is an excellent all-purpose choice.

Childbirth in Other Cultures If the midwife attending a birth in the Yucatán Peninsula is concerned about the progress of labor, a common remedy is to give the laboring woman a raw egg. The woman swallows the egg, shudders with revulsion, and regurgitates it; the heaving usually brings on powerful contractions to complete the process of labor.

notes

*Never teach your child to be cunning
for you may be certain that you will be one of the first victims of his shrewdness.*

JOSH BILLINGS

DAY	DATE:
138	*128 days to go*

If your baby is a boy, by today the testes will have begun their descent from the pelvis into the scrotum. Remember that ovaries and the testes are formed from the same tissue. The ovaries will remain in place, however.

While you may be noticing varicose veins in your legs, your rectum is also susceptible to varicose veins during pregnancy. These are called hemorrhoids and they may bleed, itch, and cause pain.

Rectal bleeding may also be caused by tears in the anus that occur because of constipation. Report any rectal bleeding to your practitioner. A medical diagnosis should be made just in case there might be another cause besides constipation.

Did You Know? The best way to prevent hemorrhoids is to avoid becoming constipated. Consult with your practitioner regarding preventative aids.

notes

DAY	DATE:
139	*127 days to go*

Even though its eyelids are fused, the baby is now making blinking movements. Much of the baby's skeleton has hardened into bone.

Your practitioner may report that your heart rate has increased somewhat during this month. That's normal and just a sign that your body is having to work a little harder to maintain the pregnancy.

Food Facts Proteins are the only substances that build tissue. Protein must be provided for the growth of the baby, placenta, uterus, and breasts, and to permit necessary increases in blood volume.

For Your Information If you prefer vegetables, pasta, and legumes to meat, you can fulfill your daily protein requirements during pregnancy by eating dried beans, peas, nuts, lima beans, barley, whole wheat bread, cornmeal, macaroni, rice, and spaghetti with tomato sauce.

When you are dealing with a child, keep all your wits about you, and sit on the floor.
AUSTIN O'MALLEY

DAY 140

DATE:

126 days to go

The size and strength of the baby's hands have improved so that by now, it can grip with some force. If your baby is a female, her uterus is completely formed and has just undergone its most rapid period of growth.

At the end of this fifth month of pregnancy, your baby measures about 7 inches (191 mm) in length and is about the size of a Barbie doll. In less than two weeks, the baby has gained more than 3½ ounces (100 g). Right now your baby weighs a little less than a pound (about 437 g). Hold a pound package of butter in your hand. That's about how much your baby weighs right now and how heavy it would feel if you could hold it.

Childbirth in Other Cultures Midwives in Sumatra cut the baby's umbilical cord with a flute to make sure the child has a good voice.

Did You Know? After birth, the baby's nose may be runny from accumulated amniotic fluid. If you didn't know this, you might think the baby had already caught a cold.

How are you feeling today?

MOOD:

ENERGY:

APPETITE:

BABY MOVEMENT?

CONTRACTIONS?

notes

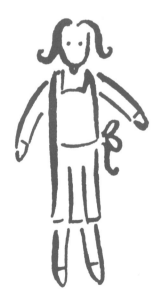

Respect the child. Be not too much his parent. Trespass not on his solitude.

RALPH WALDO EMERSON

Lunar Month 6

THINGS TO DO THIS MONTH:

Sign up for childbirth preparation classes.

Keep lotion or other moisturizers on your abdomen to minimize itching due to stretching skin.

Keep fat intake low and exercise regularly to avoid gaining unnecessary weight.

Prevent leg cramps and backache.

Change positions to improve circulation and avoid tingling sensations in your hands and feet.

Elevate your legs to reduce the likelihood of swollen feet and ankles.

Avoid urinary tract infections.

Reduce discomfort due to hemorrhoids.

Make sure your calcium and protein intake are adequate to support the baby's growing brain and skeletal system.

Monitor your sun exposure carefully and use sunscreens, hats, and protective clothing when outdoors.

week 21

DAY	DATE:
141	*125 days to go*

The bones of the middle ear (the three smallest bones in the human body: the hammer, the anvil, and the stirrup) are beginning to harden to make sound conduction possible. While the baby might be able to transmit sound information to its brain at this point in its development, it's not clear that they have any way of interpreting the sound because the brain is so immature.

You can actually feel your own cervix. It is a bump deep within the vagina. The cervical opening feels like a small indentation. Toward the end of pregnancy the cervix becomes quite difficult to feel on your own due to the changing position of the baby. You cannot reliably check your own cervical dilation in the third trimester and should not attempt to do so.

For Your Information In the weeks and months ahead, some parents will go to great lengths to offer auditory stimulation to their babies (headphones on the pregnant abdomen, speaking through a megaphone directed at the uterus to amplify sound, etc.). While it can't hurt, it might not help, either.

Food Facts If you happen to be pregnant when fresh berries are available, raw berries (like strawberries, raspberries, etc.) are a good source of vitamin C. Three-fourths of a cup of strawberries contains 66 mg of vitamin C, more than half of your day's requirement. Berries should not be washed until you are ready to eat them. They may break apart, and wet berries might become moldy much faster.

DAY	DATE:
142	*124 days to go*

The baby will gain considerable weight within the next four weeks. By Week 25, the baby will weigh almost twice as much as it does today.

Because the baby is growing so actively, your body at this point needs and stores more protein than at any other time during your pregnancy. Any varicose veins you have will tend to subside after childbirth, but each succeeding pregnancy may aggravate any existing condition.

Chart your waist size and weight here.

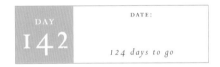

WAIST SIZE	WEIGHT

Food Facts Prepared soups can be quick and nutritious during pregnancy. Split-pea soup, New England clam chowder, pork and beans, cream of potato, and chicken noodle offer the most protein (8–9 g per 1-cup serving). Tomato-based soups, including minestrone, offer up to half of the vitamin A needed daily during pregnancy.

If you want a baby, have a new one. Don't baby the old one.
JESSAMYN WEST

Childbirth in Other Cultures If an expectant mother among the Ainu people of Northern Japan exercises during pregnancy, she is supposed to have a short labor for her reward.

DAY	DATE:
143	*123 days to go*

The first movements you feel the baby make will be caused by arm and leg activity. These first motions are called "quickening."

Quickening is a notable event for most pregnant women. Excluding ultrasound visualization, it generally marks the first time they feel they have had direct contact with their baby.

Childbirth Then and Now Almost all cultures have views on the moment when the spirit, or life force, enters a baby. Before the causes of conception were understood, people thought that babies were put directly into their mothers' wombs. Prior to that time, the children's spirits were thought to reside in natural formations, like rocks, ponds, or trees. Thus, from this perspective, all people were "children of the earth" because that was their first home. The views of Western society have varied. The Catholic Church believes the spirit of the baby enters with conception; English common law (the codes upon which our own American laws were built) felt that it enters when the mother first feels the baby move. Today, these beliefs are still debated, as people in the twentieth century ponder when life begins.

DAY	DATE:
144	*122 days to go*

The baby's respiratory system is still quite immature. Much more development must take place before the lungs can trap and transfer oxygen to the baby's bloodstream and can release carbon dioxide when the baby exhales.

As your uterus enlarges, you may notice some aching in your lower abdomen due to the stretching of the muscles and ligaments that support the uterus. The aching may be especially noticeable when you get up from a chair, change position, or get out of bed.

The pelvic pain might be sharp, but if it is occasional and not accompanied by any other symptoms, there is probably no cause for alarm.

Food Facts Sweet potatoes and yams are a terrific source of vitamin A during pregnancy. One-fourth cup of sweet potatoes yields 4,250 IU of vitamin A, nearly your whole day's requirement.

notes

....

....

....

....

....

....

....

....

....

....

I do not believe in a child world . . . I believe the child should be taught from the very first that the whole world is his world, that adult and child share one world, that all generations are needed.

PEARL S. BUCK

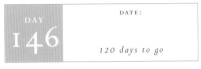

DAY 145
DATE:

121 days to go

The heat-producing brown fat that the baby has stored in its neck, chest, and crotch area will disappear shortly after birth. During months 8 and 9, white fat will be deposited under the baby's skin.

As your uterus becomes larger, you may have some concerns about having sex during pregnancy. For the most part, let your own sexual comfort be your guide. Certain positions may be more comfortable than others. Also, you may notice changes in your sexual responsiveness: for some women, it's easier to have an orgasm, for others, it's more difficult.

Since sex is part of a normal, loving relationship with your partner, sex during pregnancy is encouraged unless you are having complications, experience vaginal bleeding or fluid loss, or are having twins or multiple babies. If you have questions or concerns, check with your practitioner.

Food Facts If you're feeling hungry for something sweet and cold, opt for a Popsicle, juice bar, sherbet, sorbet, or a soft-serve cone instead of ice cream or ice milk. While ice cream can be very satisfying, it contains huge quantities of saturated fats (62 g in 1 cup of regular ice cream, 105 g in 1 cup rich ice cream, 29 g in 1 cup ice milk).

DAY 146
DATE:

120 days to go

The baby's body is becoming better proportioned. Although the head still looks large in relation to the body, the legs, arms, and trunk are not as short.

As your skin stretches, your belly may begin to itch.

For Your Comfort
Since scratching provides no relief, you may want to keep the area moist with lotion and try to prevent excessive weight gain (it will only add to your discomfort).

Childbirth Then and Now In Europe in the late 1880s, superstition played a role in assisting difficult labor. The ringing of church bells was thought to hasten delivery. A more common belief was that locks and knots in the vicinity of the pregnant woman might help with the birth. According to Pliny, the ancient Romans thought people should not cross their legs or clasp their hands near a pregnant woman.

notes

Never help a child with a task at which he feels he can succeed.
MARIA MONTESSORI

notes

DAY	DATE:
147	*119 days to go*

Fine downy lanugo covers the baby's entire body, including the head.

Your vaginal tissues will have become thicker during pregnancy, your vaginal secretions will have increased and there will be more blood in the tissues of your vagina.

IMPORTANT You, along with a coach (partner, friend, relative, etc.), should begin taking a childbirth preparation course sometime soon. Such a course will help you understand more about what will happen in the birth process and will help you involve another person who will help you concentrate on pain control through breathing, relaxation, distraction, and education. If you are giving birth at a hospital, the hospital may have its own course for expectant mothers. Even so, check with other childbirth educators in your area about course availability.

Childbirth Then and Now In colonial America the pain of labor was thought to be relieved by leaving an axe by the bed with the blade up to "cut the pain," opening the windows, or setting the horses free from the stable.

How are you feeling today?

MOOD:

ENERGY:

APPETITE:

BABY MOVEMENT?

CONTRACTIONS?

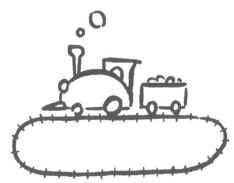

It's a great mistake, I think, to put children off with falsehoods and nonsense, when their growing powers of observation and discrimination excite in them a desire to know about things.

ANNE SULLIVAN

week 22

The baby will grow about 2 more inches (51 mm) this month to become about 14 inches (357 mm) tall. The baby's environment is becoming more crowded as it is growing and filling up the space inside the uterus.

Every day, you should become more and more aware of the baby's movement. Although the bumps and thumps are now obvious to you, it may be a few more weeks before someone else can feel the baby move by touching your abdomen.

Food Facts Excellent sources of dietary fiber include whole wheat bread, bran cereals, rye crackers, baked beans, potato crisps, pears (with skin), and peanuts.

Childbirth Then and Now Among the Chagga of what was Tanganyika, Africa, and is now Tanzania, there is a saying, "Pay attention to the pregnant woman! There is no one more important than she."

Throughout this month, changes in the appearance of your baby's skin will take place. Right now, the skin is wrinkled. When more fat is deposited and more muscle development takes place, it will begin to look smooth.

Even now your breasts are preparing for milk production and nursing. The amount of breastmilk secreted by a breastfeeding mother varies considerably from woman to woman. The average is one-half pint (235 mL) at first, increasing to a pint (470 mL) by the seventh day and two pints (940 mL) by two weeks.

Food Facts Monitor your calcium intake carefully. The easiest way to get a quick dose of calcium is to drink a glass of milk.

Childbirth in Other Cultures Salt and sweet things are forbidden to the Jivaro women of Ecuador when they're pregnant, in the belief that this deprivation will prevent the fetus from growing too big.

Besides its wrinkled appearance, the baby's skin also is transparent because it's so thin. Thus, at this time, if you could see the baby, the bones, organs, and blood vessels would be visible, as they lie just beneath the skin.

Leg cramps can be prevented by making dietary changes (adding calcium, reducing phosphorus), sitting with feet elevated rather than standing, and wearing support stockings. If you do experience a cramp in your calf muscle, stand in a lunge position (the uncramped leg should be in the lead). Press the heel of your back leg (the one that's cramped) slowly to the floor. You should feel your

Never say [to younger people] "that was before your time," because the last full moon was before their time.
BILL COSBY

muscle begin to stretch out, and the cramp should disappear. Remember not to bounce—you want a slow stretch; bouncing might injure the muscle.

For Your Health Sea salt does not contain iodine. Iodized table salt contains the trace amounts of iodine needed daily during pregnancy.

Childbirth Then and Now According to Thomas Raynalde in *The Byrthe of Mankynde* (1540): "The thynges which helpe the byrthe and make it more easie, are these. First, the woman that laboureth must eyther sytte grovelyng or els upright, leaning backwards, according as it shal seeme commodius and necessary to the partie, or as she is accustomed."

DAY	DATE:
1 5 1	*115 days to go*

 The baby continues to grow at a steady pace. More than 6 ounces (168 g) of weight will be gained during this week alone.

Like last month, you may notice aching in the small of your back.

For Your Health Take steps to prevent backache. Lying down, having a massage, and heating the area may soothe aching muscles.

Food Facts Potatoes are rich in vitamin C. One small baked potato yields 15 mg, about 15% of your day's requirement. Reduce vitamin C loss during cooking by leaving the peel on. Remove the peel (if necessary) after cooking.

DAY	DATE:
1 5 2	*114 days to go*

Most of the weight gained during this time in your baby's development is muscle and bone mass and weight increases from growing organs and tissues. Very little fat is being manufactured at this time.

As your baby grows, so do you. On average, expect to gain about a pound a week during this month.

Did You Know? The first true bonelike formation occurs in the baby's breastbone.

Parenting Tips Premoistened baby wipes are useful for cleaning baby's bottom, but there are lots of alternatives. Make your own inexpensive wipes by soaking small, unbleached paper napkins in baby oil in a shallow bowl. Store them in a covered container. Keep a roll of toilet paper or a box of tissues handy at the changing table for cleanups. Wipe a soiled bottom clean with baby oil on a cotton ball. If you use washcloths for cleanup, keep the ones used for diaper cleanup separate from the ones used for the bath.

How are you feeling today?

MOOD: ....

ENERGY: ....

APPETITE: ....

BABY MOVEMENT? ....

CONTRACTIONS? ....

Babies do not want to hear about babies; they like to be told of giants and castles, and of somewhat which can stretch and stimulate their little minds.

SAMUEL JOHNSON

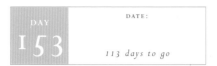

DAY
153

DATE:

113 days to go

Sounds that are heard daily by your baby include the beating of your heart, the sound of your voice resonating as you speak, the sound of air filling your lungs and being exhaled, and the growling noises made by your stomach and intestines.

As the baby's heartbeat becomes louder, it may be possible to hear the baby's heart by placing an ear to your abdomen. With a stethoscope, the baby's heartbeat can be heard well.

Did You Know? Taste buds are formed in abundance on your baby's tongue and inside its cheeks. In humans, taste buds begin to diminish in number after birth and never increase again.

Parenting Tips Sew two bath towels together to cover your changing pad or slip the pad into a pillowcase, which can be removed and laundered easily.

Your health may become impaired if vomiting connected with morning sickness persists throughout the day. Notify your practitioner immediatly if you vomit more than two or three times in a day or if you begin vomiting when you haven't before.

Parenting Tips After having a baby, someone who was with you during delivery should talk to your partner and other children if you were separated from them. Young children, especially, may be worried about your health and well-being. They will need emotional reassurance and will probably have a lot of pressing questions. After you go home, expect immature, babylike behavior from older children—a common, though temporary, response to the birth of a new sibling. It's often a signal that a child needs extra loving attention.

notes

....
....
....
....
....
....
....
....
....
....
....
....
....
....

DAY
154

DATE:

112 days to go

The baby measures 8¼ inches (210 mm) and weighs about 1⅓ pounds (598.5 g).

Today marks the completion of twenty-two weeks of pregnancy. At this point, being pregnant is nothing new—it's become a way of life! If you are still experiencing some stomach upset and nausea, eating an easily digested snack every two hours may help you feel less nauseous.

Remember, when they have a tantrum, don't have one of your own.
Dr. Judith Kuriansky

week 23

DAY
155

DATE:

111 days to go

The smallest blood vessels of the body—the capillaries—are beginning to develop under the baby's skin. As blood fills these new vessels, they give the baby's skin a red or pinkish appearance, because the blood in the capillaries is visible.

You may notice tingling sensations in your hands and feet from time to time. The cause is unknown, but changing positions may bring some relief.

Childbirth in Other Cultures When the Taureg women of the Sahara go into labor, they walk up and down the small, sandy hills of their region, returning to their hut when it's time to deliver their babies.

Parenting Tips Keep a thermos of warm water near the changing table at night for quick cleanups. You'll avoid stumbling around in the dark and having to run the tap water to get the right temperature.

DAY
156

DATE:

110 days to go

The baby continues to practice reflex movements that will be essential to its survival after birth. Its lips and mouth are sensitive, and if the baby's hand floats near its mouth, it may suck its thumb or fingers.

Even though you are probably eating well, you may still experience periodic indigestion, heartburn, bloating, and intestinal gas. These problems can be expected as your muscles relax under the influence of the pregnancy hormones. Continue to eat things that are easy to digest.

Childbirth in Other Cultures After giving birth, a Tarong woman of the Philippines is given a tea made from her charred placenta and a root that is eaten to eliminate "bad air." She is also given a cigar to smoke.

Parenting Tips If you put powder on your baby after bathing it, put the powder in your hand first and away from the baby's face, so it isn't inhaled by the baby. Don't let an older baby play with an open powder container, since some of the powder can escape and be inhaled into their lungs.

notes

It is better to bind your children to you by a feeling of respect, and by gentleness, than by fear.
TERENCE

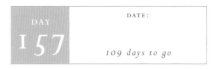

DAY
1 **57**

DATE:

109 days to go

The baby will develop a strong grip during this month—far more powerful than that of the infant soon after birth.

Mild swelling in your ankles and feet is common and expected.

Contact your practitioner if you have severe swelling. Elevate your legs whenever possible. It's important to rest.

Parenting Tips Keep a roll of masking tape handy to mend torn tabs on disposable diapers and to mend plastic pants.

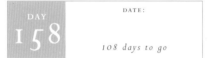

DAY
1 **58**

DATE:

108 days to go

Gradually, the baby's fingernails and toenails lengthen. They are growing from the nail beds and are beginning to cover the nail itself.

Continue to prevent urinary tract infection by drinking plenty of fluids (water and juices high in vitamin C; avoid caffeine-containing beverages), thoroughly emptying your bladder when you urinate, minimizing stress, and practicing good hygiene (shower daily and wash the vaginal area thoroughly).

Childbirth Then and Now The custom among most Native American women in the past was to deliver babies in an isolated setting, often along the banks of a stream. The Sioux woman sat with her legs crossed at the ankle and her thighs separated. Her arms were crossed over her chest, her head was bowed, and her body was bent forward, especially during contractions. It's interesting to note that ancient Egyptian drawings show women in this same cross-legged position, seemingly in the act of giving birth.

Parenting Tips You won't be giving your baby a full bath until the umbilical cord falls off. It takes a week or two for the stump of the umbilical cord to dry up and drop off, leaving the healed scar we call the navel. Even then, remember that, until it starts crawling, only baby's bottom, face, and neck will get dirty. First babies probably get bathed more than later-born children because parents have more time than they do with two or more children. A day without a bath is not a disgrace, provided the dirty spots have been wiped clean. On the other hand, a bath can be relaxing for both of you.

notes

Don't demand respect as a parent. Demand civility and insist on honesty.
But respect is something you must earn—with kids as well as with adults.
WILLIAM ATTWOOD

DAY	DATE:
159	*107 days to go*

Over the next three days, blood vessels will develop in the baby's lungs.

If you have hemorrhoids, you may experience some rectal bleeding in addition to the usual symptoms of pain and itching.

Did You Know? Prevention is still the key for treating hemorrhoids: drink plenty of fluids, eat fresh fruits and vegetables in quantity, avoid sitting in place for hours at a time, exercise moderately, and walk to reduce or minimize their development.

Chart your waist size and weight here.

WAIST SIZE   WEIGHT
....

Parenting Tips If you're ever in a situation where you have to give a refrigerator-cold bottle to a hungry baby, don't worry. It's not harmful in any way. The baby can digest cold formula just as well as warm formula, it's just not as appealing.

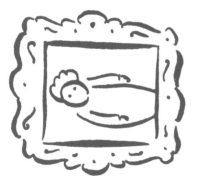

DAY	DATE:
160	*106 days to go*

The baby's nostrils (which until now have been plugged) begin to open. By today, blood vessels will have developed in the lungs. After birth, these vessels will allow blood to flow through the lungs to intercept oxygen and circulate it to the baby's tissues.

The amniotic fluid that surrounds the baby is removed and replaced by your system every three hours. This means the total daily exchange is equivalent to six gallons (25.6 L) in volume.

Did You Know? The main sources of incoming amniotic fluid appear to be the baby's own lungs and kidneys. The secondary source is the amniotic sac itself. The living skin cells of the amniotic sac also produce some fluid.

Childbirth in Other Cultures For Mayan women in the Yucatán Peninsula, some pain is an expected part of birth, as it is an accepted part of life in general. No attempt is made to protect the pregnant woman by withholding information about labor and childbirth. Pain appears in the stories women tell about their own birth experiences. The storyteller makes it clear that the laboring woman's distress is normal and that her suffering will pass, just as it did for other women.

The most important thing a father can do for his children is to love their mother.
THEODORE HESBURGH

DAY 161	DATE:
	105 days to go

During this month, the buds for the baby's permanent teeth will come in, high in the gums behind the baby teeth. The baby's spine will be made up of 33 rings, 150 joints, and 1,000 ligaments, all of which are used to support its body weight. All of those structures will begin to form during this month.

Between 20 and 50% of all pregnant women develop hemorrhoids and may experience some rectal bleeding. While rectal bleeding does not signal a problem with the baby, it should be reported to your practitioner for evaluation.

Childbirth in Other Cultures The home was and is the primary place of birth among tribal peoples. The second most common place was the birthing hut, a place designated for birth alone or shared with menstruating women. Worldwide, 98% of people alive today were born at home.

Parenting Tips Help your baby avoid diaper rash by not using plastic overpants. These hold moisture in and prevent evaporation.

How are you feeling today?

MOOD:

ENERGY:

APPETITE:

BABY MOVEMENT?

CONTRACTIONS?

notes

Let your children go if you want to keep them.
MALCOLM FORBES

week 24

DAY	DATE:
162	*104 days to go*

Now that the baby's nostrils have begun to open, the baby will make muscular breathing movements as its body prepares to draw air into the lungs at birth.

You may have to adjust your schedule so you get sufficient rest.

Did You Know? From Week 15 through Week 28, the amniotic fluid volume increases at an average rate of 4½ cups minus two teaspoons (50 mL) per week, twice the weekly fluid increase during the first fifteen weeks of pregnancy.

Parenting Tips Don't be afraid to take some time alone for yourself after your baby is born. Disconnect the phone if you don't want to answer it, or let the phone machine answer it for you. Also, put a "Do Not Disturb" sign on your front door when you feel you need to.

DAY	DATE:
163	*103 days to go*

Within the next two days, air sacs (alveoli) will have developed in the baby's lungs.

By keeping your fat intake low, you will gain what weight you need to sustain your pregnancy without padding your body with fat. Avoid butter and margarine, fried foods, high calorie salad dressing, sauces and gravies, and rich desserts.

Did You Know? Animal fat (from beef, chicken, etc.) also contains vitamins A and D. Even so, fat should be eaten sparingly.

Parenting Tips Keep a rubber spatula on your changing table to apply petroleum jelly or another moisture barrier to your child's bottom. It will help to keep your hands clean and avoid problems with adhesive strips on disposable diapers not sticking.

DAY	DATE:
164	*102 days to go*

During this week, the baby's lungs will begin to secrete surfactant, a substance which keeps the lung tissue from sticking to itself.

Monitor your sun exposure carefully. Any changes you are experiencing in your skin's pigmentation (especially blotchiness) will be darkened by sun exposure. Sunscreens, hats, and light, long-sleeved clothing offer you the best protection.

*By the time the youngest children have learned to keep the house tidy,
the oldest grandchildren are on hand to tear it to pieces.*

CHRISTOPHER MORLEY

Childbirth Then and Now In rural America during the eighteenth century, the birth attendant was paid with whatever the family could afford—chickens, a twist of tobacco, or day work. Sometimes in lieu of payment, a girl child would bear the attendant's name.

Parenting Tips Invest in a rocking chair. Wood, metal, and upholstered styles are available. Rocking a baby will soothe it, will relax you, and is reported to be helpful in relieving some of the discomforts following Cesarean section. (For C-section benefit, rock sixty or more minutes per day.)

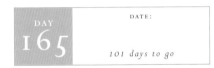

DAY
165

DATE:

101 days to go

Over the next four days, brain wave activity will begin for the baby's visual and auditory systems. The baby's sensory systems are developing the kind of connections with the brain that will be useful for interpreting input after birth. While the presence of brain wave activity indicates that the baby's eyes have encountered a light source or that the baby's ears have intercepted a sound message, no comprehension is possible yet. This system needs practice just like all the others.

Take it slow and easy when you exercise. The no pain-no gain exercise philosophy doesn't work during pregnancy. Concentrate on stretching, relaxing, and toning; avoid bouncing and strenuous workouts.

Be sure your exercises are designed for pregnant women. When in doubt, check with your practitioner.

Parenting Tips To avoid becoming disconnected with your partner, dedicate a part of every day to being together. Take a walk together, share a luncheon phone call, plan a late dinner, or whatever. The "couple" part of your relationship needs to be maintained, even though now you will soon be a family.

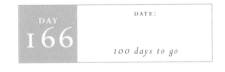

DAY
166

DATE:

100 days to go

Over the next couple of days, the baby's fingernails will become noticeable.

While the baby's nails are growing, yours may be growing well, too. Strong, long, healthy nails often accompany pregnancy because of improvements in circulation and metabolism.

Childbirth in Other Cultures The amount of recuperation time after childbirth varies considerably among different cultures. A well-to-do Goajiro Indian woman of Colombia will rest in bed for a month after delivering her first baby. Among the Yahgan of Tierra del Fuego, a new mother is back gathering shellfish with her tribe less than a day after giving birth.

Parenting Tips Help your new baby follow a predictable routine. Once established, your baby's routine, like that of the other family members, should be respected. For example, it's disruptive to wake the baby up from a scheduled (and needed) nap just because a friend or relative is visiting and wants to see the baby. It's nice for people to be interested in the newborn, but it's easier for adults to wait until the baby is ready to see them than for the baby to have to conform to the social needs of adults.

Home is not where you live but where they understand you.
CHRISTIAN MORGENSTERN

DAY

167

DATE:

99 days to go

The baby is still lean—its skin wrinkles while covering its nearly fat-free body.

For the sake of your circulation, remember to change position frequently. Optimal circulation to the placenta and fetus is possible when you lie on your left side.

For Your Comfort Avoid standing in a fixed position, if at all possible. If you do stand, do so briefly while resting one foot on a footstool. Sit with feet elevated or lie down when you can.

Parenting Tips Don't worry if you don't feel overwhelming love for your baby from the moment of birth. Early feelings for a baby can be remarkably ambivalent sometimes. Parental love often takes weeks and sometimes months to develop, so enjoy getting to know one another and developing a lasting parent-child bond.

It's important to monitor your blood pressure during pregnancy for signs of elevation. Blood pressure increases are most common after Week 20, and affect about 7% of all pregnant women. Increased blood pressure that is accompanied by edema is called preeclampsia; the more severe form of high blood pressure during pregnancy is called eclampsia. (The older term for both of these conditions was toxemia of pregnancy.)

Did You Know? The baby's skin will contain more than 500,000 hair follicles at birth; they begin forming during this month.

notes

....
....
....
....
....
....
....
....
....
....
....

DAY

168

DATE:

98 days to go

This was an important month in the baby's life. At this point, it has completed two-thirds of its stay in your womb. In the next three months, the baby will be progressively able to survive without such an intimate attachment. By the end of this sixth month of pregnancy, your baby will measure at least 9 inches long (230 mm) and weigh at least 1¾ pounds (779 g).

How are you feeling today?

MOOD: ....

ENERGY: ....

APPETITE: ....

BABY MOVEMENT? ....

CONTRACTIONS? ....

Insanity is hereditary; you get it from your children.

SAM LEVENSON

Lunar Month 7

THINGS TO DO THIS MONTH:

Rest to reduce fatigue, pain in your pelvis, inner thighs, and groin area.

Monitor your baby's movement by "counting the kicks."

Soothe skin irritation due to trapped perspiration by applying lotions, powders, and keeping your pelvic area and the area under your breasts clean and dry.

Take precautions to prevent fainting, reduce swelling (edema) in your hands and feet, and prevent or minimize the effect of varicose veins.

Avoid bladder leakage and manage shortness of breath.

Relieve pain and tenderness in the rib area right below your breasts.

Shift positions to release feelings of pressure when lying down.

Add about 300 extra calories per day to your diet during these last months of pregnancy.

Contact your practitioner immediately if you have severe headaches; blurry vision; sudden weight gain; severe swelling in the hands, feet, ankles, and/or face; or vaginal itching and changes in discharge.

Check with your practitioner before you plan a trip that involves air travel.

week 25

DAY 169	DATE:
	97 *days to go*

By the end of this week, the baby will grow about ½ inch (12.7 mm) longer.

As the baby grows, the amniotic sac grows, too. It is always a closed bubble and forms a water-tight seal around the umbilical cord, which protrudes through it.

Childbirth Then and Now Many women kneel during labor, resting their upper bodies on a chair, tree stump, or on their own arms and elbows. This labor position was referred to in the Bible and by Roman poets, was used in Germany during the Middle Ages, and was popular among Native North American tribal women.

Parenting Tips Parents are often concerned that their babies will get too cold or too hot when they sleep. You can test to see if your baby is cozy by touching the back of its neck. (Be sure your hand is not cold. Warm your hands under warm water first.) If the baby's neck is warm and dry, it is at a comfortable temperature. If the back of its neck is damp, it may be too hot. If its neck is cool, you might want to add a blanket. Don't use the temperature of the baby's hands or feet as a guide. They are usually cool no matter what the temperature of the rest of the baby's body is.

DAY 170	DATE:
	96 *days to go*

If your baby is a boy, sometime within the next three months, his testes will have completely descended.

If you have diabetes, your baby will begin to put on more weight than normal from this point on. (Diabetes is a condition where the pancreas doesn't produce as much insulin as needed in the body to utilize sugars for energy.) Some women begin their pregnancies with diabetes; other women can develop gestational diabetes during their pregnancies. Gestational diabetes generally clears up after the baby is born.

Chart your waist size and weight here.

WAIST SIZE	WEIGHT

Childbirth in Other Cultures The Bukinon of Mindanao in the Philippines consider the placenta to be "the brother" of the baby. They bury the placenta under the house and believe that the spirit of the placenta returns to the sky.

Parenting Tips Babies will nurse or bottle-feed until they are full. Don't start urging bottle-fed babies to finish the bottle or you will risk training them to overeat. A newborn's stomach is only about the size of its little fist, so your baby will need to feed often and in relatively small amounts at first.

A child is a curly, dimpled lunatic.
RALPH WALDO EMERSON

DAY 171	DATE:
	95 *days to go*

The baby's lungs continue their rapid growth.

You will need about an extra 300 calories per day now, as you enter the last three months of your pregnancy. Nonpregnant adults can generally maintain their weight and good health on 2,100 calories per day, but pregnant women generally require about 2,400 calories a day.

TIME TO REFLECT   *This week marks the beginning of your third—and last—trimester of pregnancy. As you look back on your baby's growth and your pregnancy experience so far, what are some of the moments you remember best?*

Parenting Tips When you hold your baby to your shoulder to burp it after a feeding, put a diaper on your shoulder to catch dribbles. If you're not comfortable holding the baby at your shoulder, try laying it on your lap, tummy down with its head turned a little to the side. Rub its back from the bottom up or pat gently. You can also burp a baby by sitting it on your lap, placing a hand on its chest, and leaning it forward while gently rubbing its back.

notes

There are times when parenthood seems nothing but feeding the mouth that bites you.
PETER DE VRIES

DAY	DATE:
172	94 *days to go*

The baby's brain continues its rapid growth.

You may notice some vaginal itching periodically. Vaginal itching may be due to a yeast infection or lack of regular hygiene (cleansing with mild, nondrying soap and water or with unscented mineral oil). It is also one of the symptoms associated with gestational diabetes.

Childbirth in Other Cultures The Alor women of Indonesia return to work in the fields ten days after their babies are born. During the day, they leave their babies in the care of relatives, they breast-feed the baby as soon as they come in from the fields, and they sleep with their babies at night.

Parenting Tips If you plan to breast-feed your baby, have several pillows available so you can experiment with the most comfortable arrangement for the two of you. You might find that placing the baby on a pillow on your lap puts it at just the right level for nursing. You may want to rest your nursing arm on a pillow while the baby is feeding. If you nurse in bed, you may want several pillows to rest on or a bed pillow with arms for comfort.

DAY	DATE:
173	93 *days to go*

By this time, the baby's brain wave patterns are similar to those of a full term baby at birth. Activity is beginning in the portions of the brain that process visual and auditory information.

Automobile driving may be continued until your size makes you uncomfortable or restricts your movement. The shoulder strap shouldn't be uncomfortable. Push the lap belt under your tummy if you wish. Until that time, take all the same safety precautions you would at any other time: wear your seatbelt every time you drive, never drive while "in a hurry" or when you're distracted, stay within the speed limit, and drive defensively, watching out for other motorists.

For Your Health Protein is fundamental to any woman's diet during pregnancy. Eight ounces (224 g) of protein are generally recommended: the sources can be eggs, fish, chicken, pork, nuts, dairy products, or legumes.

Parenting Tips While it isn't critical for development, some parents hold their babies in one arm for one bottle feeding and in the other arm for the next so the baby can practice looking to the left and to the right.

Having a family is like having a bowling alley installed in your brain.
MARTIN MULL

DAY 174	DATE:
	92 *days to go*

During this month, the forebrain (portion of the baby's brain just behind the forehead) will enlarge to cover all other developed brain structures, while still maintaining its hemisphere divisions. As a result, some significant brain developments will occur.

As your baby grows physically stronger, its thumping and bumping will become stronger, too. You can monitor your baby's movement by counting its kicks. At least ten kicks should be felt within a two-hour period (the best time to count is between 7 and 10 P.M. when the baby is most likely to be active).

 Let your practitioner know if your baby kicks fewer times than ten.

Parenting Tips If you're bottlefeeding, shake the formula in the bottle to distribute the warmed milk evenly. Test the temperature of the bottled milk by squirting a drop or two on your inside wrist. If the milk feels comfortably warm, it's the right temperature for the baby.

DAY 175	DATE:
	91 *days to go*

The baby has grown ½ inch (13 mm) in just 7 days.

As the baby gets bigger, you may notice some shortness of breath. As your growing uterus presses on your diaphragm, it becomes harder to fill your lungs and to breathe out completely.

IMPORTANT To help manage this breathlessness, slow down, minimize stress, and reduce your activity level.

Parenting Tips Store baby bottles in the refrigerator in an empty cardboard six-pack bottle holder to keep them together and prevent them from tipping over.

notes

Children are a real comfort in your old age—and they make you reach it sooner, too.
JAMES COX

week 26

DAY	DATE:
176	*90 days to go*

The baby's muscle tone is gradually improving. Its hands can grip with some strength now.

As your growing baby becomes more and more active, you may notice that your sleep is sometimes interrupted by its restlessness.

Childbirth in Other Cultures The Pawnee women of North America and women of West Micronesia squat during labor, resting their backs against the back of a birth assistant or their mother for support and resistance.

Parenting Tips If you're planning to breast-feed, it's a good idea to take a front-buttoning nightgown or pajama with you to the hospital or birth center or have one available to put on after homebirth. This style is much more convenient and accessible than back-buttoning or pullover styles. If you plan to nurse the baby in your bed, you'll want to buy a crib-sized waterproof protector to keep sheets and blankets from getting damp.

DAY	DATE:
177	*89 days to go*

By now, the baby's body is composed of 2–3% body fat.

From time to time, you might experience some pelvic pain as your uterus grows and stretches the ligaments. Most often, the pain is felt in the groin area and inside your thighs, especially after you walk or exercise. Resting should bring you some relief.

Childbirth in Other Cultures The Siriono women of Bolivia give birth in a hut crowded with other women, but no one offers any help. The laboring woman rests in a hammock slung low to the ground, and when it is born, the baby is actually allowed to slip out of the hammock and onto the ground, ostensibly to encourage it to breathe.

Parenting Tips If bottle-feeding, use denture cleanser tablets to clean glass baby bottles. Let the bottles soak according to directions (usually a half hour), then brush with a bottle brush and rinse.

notes

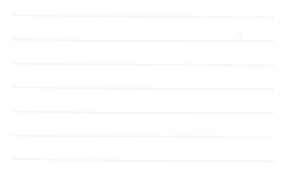

It is the child in man that is the source of his uniqueness and creativeness.
ERIC HOFFER

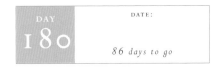

DAY 178

DATE:

88 days to go

The baby's eyelids unfuse and open.

Sometimes perspiration trapped in the folds of your skin can irritate the skin. Such irritation is most noticeable in the pelvic area and under your breasts. Lotions and powders may feel soothing; also, use good hygiene and keep the area extra clean.

Childbirth in Other Cultures African Hottentot women move very little during labor. They are packed into a small hut crowded with other women and can barely find room to give birth.

Parenting Tips If you're bottle-feeding, open and invert your vegetable steamer basket to clean or sterilize baby bottles, nipples, and rings in boiling water. The steamer keeps all the pieces together and takes up less room than the loose pieces in a big pot.

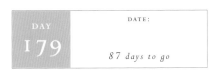

DAY 179

DATE:

87 days to go

In the next day or so, the baby's eyes will be completely formed.

You may have more swelling (edema) in your hands and feet now.

IMPORTANT Avoid standing. Rest with your legs elevated. Avoid very salty foods. All of these precautions will reduce swelling.

Parenting Tips If bottle-feeding, rinse out empty bottles as soon as possible or you'll find "cottage cheese" in them. To get rid of the sour-milk smell, fill bottles with warm water, add a teaspoon of baking soda, shake well, and let them stand overnight.

DAY 180

DATE:

86 days to go

The baby's sucking and swallowing skills are improving.

During pregnancy, a number of conditions can cause fainting: particularly hot weather, sudden changes in posture, standing for long periods of time, fatigue or excitement, stuffy rooms, and crowds.

Childbirth in Other Cultures In most cultures, older women are responsible for attending women during childbirth. Some cultures designate certain women to be midwives; others assign the task to female relatives. Men are usually not allowed in the room with the laboring woman.

Parenting Tips If bottle-feeding, regulate the flow of bottled milk by loosening the bottle collar if the flow is too slow or tightening it if the flow is too fast. If you need to enlarge the hole in the nipple, put a toothpick in the hole and boil the nipple for three minutes. Take care that the hole doesn't get too big.

It is a wise child that knows his own father.
HOMER

DAY	DATE:
181	*85 days to go*

Today is a very significant day: your baby's lungs are now capable of breathing air.

Now that your baby can breathe air, you can breathe a sigh of relief! Should your baby be born before its due date, it will have a much easier time breathing by itself and adapting to the outside world.

Did You Know? At birth, a major valve must close inside the baby's heart to keep the used blood and the fresh, oxygenated blood separated.

Parenting Tips You might want to prepare a snack for yourself to accompany the baby's nighttime feedings. (Baby may not be the only one who's hungry!)

notes

DAY	DATE:
182	*84 days to go*

Today, as Week 26 comes to a close, your baby measures almost 10 inches (254 mm) in length and weighs 2⅛ pounds (952 g). In just two weeks, your baby has gained 6 ounces (168 g) and has grown ¾ inch (19.1 mm).

Your uterus continues to push on your bladder, reducing its capacity. During pregnancy, the tubes that lead from the kidneys to the bladder lack tone and are more readily dilated, kinked, and compressed. Thus, even with a smaller capacity, the bladder can't be emptied as efficiently and urinary tract infection can result.

For Your Comfort
Since the muscles of your pelvic floor may not be able to prevent leakage when you laugh, cough, or strain to lift something, empty your bladder often.

Parenting Tips If you're bottlefeeding, you can boil nipples and glass bottles in water in a glass jar or bowl in the microwave or on the stovetop to clean them. Add a teaspoon of vinegar to the water to prevent hard-water deposits from forming in the boiling jar.

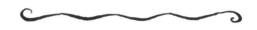

How are you feeling today?

Mood:

Energy:

Appetite:

Baby Movement?

Contractions?

It is a wise father that knows his own child.
WILLIAM SHAKESPEARE

week 27

	DATE:
DAY **183**	*83 days to go*

By today, there are eyelashes present on your baby's eyelids. Your baby's eyes are sensitive to various levels of light and darkness, but can't detect objects yet. Since the light waves of the visible spectrum carry visual information to your baby's brain, the baby's eyes are preparing to see after birth.

Pregnancy is one of the three periods in a woman's life when there seems to be a lowering of the ability to cope with the emotional experiences of life. The other two times are at puberty and menopause. There is much individual variation from woman to woman; biological (i.e., hormonal), social, and psychological factors influence emotional reactivity.

Chart your waist size and weight here.

WAIST SIZE .... WEIGHT ....

Parenting Tips If you're planning to breast-feed, one of the most important things you'll need to do is learn to relax. Relaxation will allow your milk to flow. Select a quiet place to breast-feed. Be sure it is free from distractions (and without a clock to make you feel rushed). The baby will stop nursing when it is full. Sometimes feeding sessions take a little longer and sometimes they move a little more quickly. It will be unpredictable at first.

	DATE:
DAY **184**	*82 days to go*

This is another highly significant day in your baby's development. The baby's brain can now direct rhythmic breathing and control body temperature.

This means that if your baby is born now, its brain can stimulate it to breathe and sustain that activity without medical intervention (i.e., the baby is now "viable"). It also means that the baby's body can help regulate its own temperature, taking steps to cool down when too warm or warm up when too cold.

Childbirth in Other Cultures In most cultures, a new mother is encouraged to nurse her baby right away. In some, however, first feeding is delayed for two or three days because of the belief that the first milk, or colostrum, is dangerous. Until the mother's milk comes in, the baby is given herbal tea or soft food.

Parenting Tips If your baby doesn't like holding a bottle filled with cold juice or milk, slip a small sock over the bottle to keep its hands warmer.

Thou shalt not belittle your child.
FITZHUGH DODSON

DAY
185

DATE:

81 days to go

Each day that passes brings the baby closer to birth and closer to completing the prenatal phase of their development. The baby's ability to thrive outside your womb improves with each passing day.

Your uterus will go from weighing 2 ounces (56 g) to nearly 2.2 pounds (986 g) by the end of your pregnancy. This month your weekly weight gain should taper off to ¾ pound (336 g) and then next month to ½ pound (224 g).

Childbirth in Other Cultures Among the peoples living in the Yucatán Peninsula, the woman's husband is expected to be present during her labor and childbirth. The culture says he should see how a woman suffers. This rule is quite stringent, and absent husbands are blamed for poor birth outcomes.

Parenting Tips The lids from Heinz strained baby juices fit on Evenflo baby bottles.

DAY
186

DATE:

80 days to go

Over the next three days or so, the baby's skin will begin to be smoother as more fat is deposited underneath its surface.

Your blood pressure may begin to rise somewhat during this month. Slight increases are considered normal.

Contact your practitioner immediately if you experience severe headaches, blurry vision, sudden weight gain, or severe swelling in the hands, feet, ankles, or face. These symptoms can indicate high blood pressure which can be dangerous for both you and your baby.

Parenting Tips A can of baby formula can be sealed with a plastic pet food lid before refrigerating.

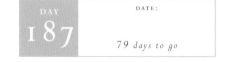

DAY
187

DATE:

79 days to go

Over the next three days, the baby will become more sensitive to light, sound, taste, and smell. The touch sensitivity of your baby's skin is already well established.

Your baby's body is preparing to see you, hear your voice, recognize you by your distinctive smell, and taste the liquid nutrition you will provide. Imagine what you will say to your baby when the two of you meet and how you will stroke its skin and hold its tiny hand. Your baby's birth is not very far away.

Did You Know? Each square inch of the baby's skin will ultimately contain 700 sweat glands, 100 oil-bearing glands, and 21,000 cells sensitive to heat.

Parenting Tips Wash baby bottles in the dishwasher if you have one. They won't need to be sterilized afterward. To keep nipples, caps, and bottle rings together, place them all in a laundry bag (the mesh bags used to wash delicate clothing).

The world talks to the mind. Parents speak more intimately—they talk to the heart.
Haim Ginott

DAY	DATE:
188	78 days to go

By today, the surface of the baby's skin is smoother and whiter as body fat accumulates under its surface. The fat the baby is putting on is white fat, not the brown fat that is used in temperature regulation earlier in the pregnancy. White fat is insulating and is an energy source. Fat babies aren't necessarily healthier babies, but some fat is needed for normal body functioning.

The bladder is usually a convex (rounded) organ, but is rendered concave (squashed) from external pressure during pregnancy. Thus, its retention capacity is greatly reduced.

Childbirth in Other Cultures Aymara mothers of Brazil take their new babies with them wherever they go. They also sleep with their babies for the first two years of life.

notes

....

....

....

....

....

....

....

....

....

....

....

....

DAY	DATE:
189	77 days to go

The baby's eyes can now move in their sockets. The baby is practicing looking.

What does the baby see? Imagine, for a moment, what the inside of the womb must look like. Under bright lights or sunlight and without the protection of your clothing, the baby's world might look pinkish, as the light shines through your vessels. At night, with clothing, or in a darkened room, it must be dark. The baby is probably aware of changes in light intensity. But "pink" is a stimulus that will take months to perceive, since even at birth, the baby's color-vision apparatus seems to distinguish only among pure reds, greens, and yellows.

Childbirth in Other Cultures In many cultures there are taboos against intercourse during the time of breast-feeding. Among the Arapesh of New Guinea, intercourse is forbidden until the baby takes its first steps.

Parenting Tips Help the baby ease off to sleep at night by bathing it just before bedtime. A bath will help to warm and relax it.

How are you feeling today?

MOOD: ....

ENERGY: ....

APPETITE: ....

BABY MOVEMENT? ....

CONTRACTIONS? ....

I honestly feel the less parents know and the more they are and try to be, the better off their kids will be.
ROBERT COLE

week 28

DAY	DATE:
190	*76 days to go*

Within the next three days, the baby's brain begins to take on a wrinkled appearance because of its rapid growth. The wrinkling of the surface of the brain is normal and necessary. The wrinkles are called convolutions. A convoluted brain contains more brain cells than a smooth, nonconvoluted brain and is potentially more powerful.

Varicose veins during pregnancy result from the increased blood flow to the uterus which slows blood return from the lower limbs.

Childbirth in Other Cultures In Southeast Asia, a fire is lit in the birthing hut to "roast," or "smoke," the new mother. The heat and smoke from the fire are thought to reduce soreness and to prevent the uterus from falling.

Parenting Tips Warm the baby's bottom sheet with a heating pad or a hot-water bottle before you lay the baby down to sleep. A cold bed may have a jarring effect. Don't use an electric blanket or heating pad as the baby's blanket, though. The electrical cords and electricity can be hazardous.

IMPORTANT Never put an infant down for a nap on a waterbed, leave a baby on a waterbed unattended, or sleep with a baby on a waterbed. The waterbed mattress can fold around its face and suffocate it. The baby could also get caught between the mattress and the frame.

DAY	DATE:
191	*75 days to go*

The baby will put on more than 1 pound (448 g) during this month.

During this month the baby will actively absorb and store the nutrients you make available: calcium for its developing skeleton, iron for its red blood cells, and protein for its growth.

From now on, your prenatal visits with your practitioner will take place every two weeks. It's important for your practitioner to keep tabs on how things are progressing as you come down to the final weeks.

Parenting Tips To help the baby feel secure when it sleeps, position it in one corner of the crib or bassinet, touching a bumper or soft padding.

notes

....

....

....

....

....

....

....

....

....

....

Never raise your hand to your children—it leaves your midsection unprotected.
ROBERT ORBEN

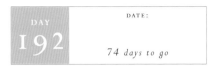

DAY 192   DATE:

74 *days to go*

 By this time, red blood cell production is entirely taken over by the bone marrow. (Remember that red blood cells were first produced by tissue groups called the blood islands; later the spleen assumes some responsibility for red blood cell production.)

Traveling by air is generally not recommended from around this time in your pregnancy until after the birth.

Contact your practitioner if you feel you must travel by air during this time.

For Your Health Air travel raises concerns about the impact of altitude changes, the dehydration caused by travel, the difficulty of sitting for such long periods of time in cramped quarters, and the distance from medical care (both on the plane and at your destination).

DAY 193   DATE:

73 *days to go*

Since the baby's eyelids are now unfused, they can open and close. Much of the time, the baby's eyes are open and the eyes are practicing "looking" movements.

You may experience some pain and tenderness in the rib area right below your breasts if the baby sits high in your uterus (pain is also due to frequent kicking).

For Your Comfort
You can relieve some of the rib area discomfort by lying down when you can and avoiding bending forward. The baby will begin to shift position and settle more into your pelvis as the pregnancy continues.

IMPORTANT Don't place a new infant face-down on a sheepskin rug, comforter, or other fluffy bedding because there is a risk of suffocation. Wait until the baby is old enough to lift and turn its head easily.

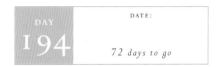

DAY 194   DATE:

72 *days to go*

The process of myelinization begins to speed nerve cell transmission. Myelin is a fatty substance that coats the outside of nerve cells and makes nerve cell transmission faster, easier, and more efficient.

When you sleep, you may notice some discomfort due to indigestion or to the pressure of the baby and your uterus on your ribs and diaphragm.

For Your Comfort
Try shifting positions to release the pressure due to indigestion and avoid eating right before bedtime. Raising the head of the bed or having an extra pillow may help.

Parenting Tips Try to establish a sleep routine from the beginning, so the baby can anticipate going to sleep at a particular time. Sing the same song each time, rub the baby in a special spot only at bedtime, rock or read to it, etc. This routine will be especially helpful when you're away from home and the baby needs to rest.

One father is more than a hundred schoolmasters.

GEORGE HERBERT

DAY 195

DATE:

71 days to go

By now, most of the lanugo (the downy hair that covered the baby's body) has disappeared except for patches on the back and shoulders.

You have probably noticed that the whitish vaginal discharge has gotten heavier. This is normal.

Contact your practitioner if the vaginal discharge is discolored or thick or is accompanied by symptoms of discomfort (pain, burning, itching), bleeding, or unusual odor.

Parenting Tips Feed the baby in as upright a position as possible. The bubble at the bottom of the baby's stomach will rise and be burped easily, preventing the pain of trapped air in its stomach.

notes

....
....
....
....
....
....
....
....
....
....
....
....
....
....
....
....

DAY 196

DATE:

70 days to go

The baby's toenails are visible, and it probably has a good head of hair by this point.

When this day ends, you will have been pregnant for seven complete months.

Did You Know? While the baby's growth has been rapid and sustained for many weeks, its growth rate will begin to slow as the date of birth approaches.

Parenting Tips Let a baby who is crying inconsolably suck a peppermint candy stick as you hold it in its mouth or melt a small piece of peppermint in water and give it in a bottle. If the baby is experiencing some stomach upset, the peppermint can have a soothing effect.

How are you feeling today?

MOOD: ....

ENERGY: ....

APPETITE: ....

BABY MOVEMENT? ....

CONTRACTIONS? ....

Blessed are the young, for they shall inherit the national debt.
HERBERT HOOVER

Lunar Month 8

THINGS TO DO THIS MONTH:

Continue with your well-balanced diet; make sure your calcium intake is sufficient.

Adjust to increased clumsiness by moving slowly and deliberately.

Reduce backache and achiness in your abdomen by staying off your feet, avoiding overexertion and fatigue, and applying dry heat.

Anticipate more frequent Braxton-Hicks contractions as your uterine muscles prepare for birth.

Avoid leg cramps and minimize edema.

Anticipate some leakage of "premilk" from your breasts.

Avoid or minimize constipation.

Relieve skin itchiness and irritation by swimming or applying lotion to the affected area.

Avoid long trips by motor vehicle (most long-distance travel is not recommended at this point in pregnancy).

Prevent dizziness, headaches, and faintness.

week 29

	DATE:
DAY **197**	
	69 days to go

 Your baby's crown-to-rump measurement is now over 10 inches (269 mm). Its weight is at least 2¾ pounds (1,232 g).

Only about 10% of women experience varicose veins during pregnancy.

Your practitioner may order more blood tests for you sometime during this month to make sure your pregnancy is progressing well.

Parenting Tips If you need to stay in bed right after the birth (as women with C-sections often do), make the bed a playpen and babycare station by keeping toys, books, diapers, clothing, and food within reach. It's important to get some temporary help with caring for the baby so you can rest and recuperate. Right after the baby is born, use disposable plates and cups to minimize cleanup.

notes

	DATE:
DAY **198**	
	68 days to go

The baby's growth in height and weight will begin to slow between now and birth. Even so, the baby will gain about two pounds (896 g) this month.

Backache may be due to poor posture or poor muscle tone, especially if you have had other children.

Chart your waist size and weight here.

WAIST SIZE	WEIGHT

Did You Know? Your baby's brain is now so sophisticated that if it was born today, it could see, hear, remember, and learn. Western scientists believe that the presence of these brain activities marks the beginning of true consciousness, since the baby's brain exhibits all of the brain waves (although not in the same sequence) that an adult brain exhibits.

Parenting Tips If you use a soft-fabric front carrier, let the infant sleep upright occasionally if you are comfortable doing so.

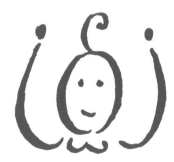

Unlike grownups, children have little need to deceive themselves.

J. W. GOETHE

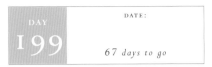

DAY 199

DATE:

67 days to go

If the baby is born now, it may have a callous on its thumb from sucking it in the womb.

Cavities in your teeth during pregnancy are more often caused by a slight decrease in the pH of the saliva or by inadequate hygiene or dental care than by any pregnancy-induced changes in the teeth themselves.

IMPORTANT While your baby isn't growing much bigger in ways that can be easily measured, its internal systems and tissues continue to become more sophisticated. For those reasons, calcium, protein, iron, and folic acid intake are more important than ever.

Parenting Tips For easy access and ease of carrying, keep baby bath items in a plastic organizer-carrier with a handle.

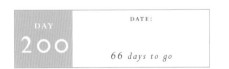

DAY 200

DATE:

66 days to go

For about the last month, the baby has assumed the fetal position in your uterus. The legs have been drawn in to the chest, because there isn't room for them to straighten out.

You will continue to notice strong, methodical activity from the baby. Sometimes it seems as though the baby is more active at night than at other times. This may be the case, but it may also be that you simply notice the movements more because you are less distracted by other things.

Childbirth in Other Cultures New mothers in Mexico are given steam baths after giving birth to help relieve pain and soreness.

Parenting Tips Keep the time that your newborn is undressed to a minimum. When the baby is older, it will become better at regulating its own body temperature. Warm a towel near a heat duct in the dryer or by a sunny window to keep the baby warm and cozy after a bath (but be sure it's not too hot!). Baby towels that are hooded in one corner also help prevent heat loss.

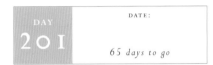

DAY 201

DATE:

65 days to go

There are four layers of tissue in the placenta separating your blood supply from the baby's. Unless some breakdown of the placenta occurs, the baby's blood does not mix with yours.

You may notice that you're a little clumsy these days. This is due to the increased size of your uterus, the loosening of your joints to prepare for childbirth, and the shifts in the baby's position.

If you fall, contact your practitioner so they can ask you about any other symptoms you might be experiencing.

Did You Know? Take care not to lose your balance but, if you do, remember that the baby is protected by one of the most efficient shock-minimizing systems on earth—the amniotic fluid contained in your tough, muscular uterus.

There are only two lasting bequests we can hope to give our children. One of these is roots, the other, wings.

HODDING CARTER

DAY
202

DATE:

64 days to go

The baby's brain is still developing rapidly, increasing the number of interconnections between individual nerve cells and identifying groups of cells that will perform complicated functions throughout the baby's lifetime.

As your uterus continues to stretch these final weeks, your abdomen will ache more.

For Your Comfort
Try to rest and get off your feet. A heating pad may help.

Parenting Tips Put the baby down when it is drowsy but still awake, so it will learn to drift off to sleep without help from you.

DAY
203

DATE:

63 days to go

Sometime between now and birth, the baby's testes will have completely descended if it's a boy. The testes are formed in the body cavity from the same tissue that forms the female baby's ovaries. While the female's ovaries stay in place, the body cavity is too warm for the male's testes and their immature sperm-producing mechanisms. Eventually, the testes migrate into the scrotum. In the scrotum, the tissue of the temperature-sensitive testes can be perfectly maintained by bringing the testes closer to the body to warm them or relaxing the muscles to distance them from the body and cool them.

Calcium needs are greatest during the last twelve weeks of your pregnancy, when rapid ossification of the baby's skeleton is taking place and calcium is required for bone development. The calcium in milk or milk products is very readily absorbed and utilized, while the calcium in pill form is not.

Did You Know? A total of 222 bones is needed to adequately support the soft parts of the baby's body, especially during sitting and standing.

Parenting Tips Cover your bassinet pad with a standard pillow case. When a fresh side is needed, just flip it over.

notes

....

....

....

....

....

....

....

....

....

How are you feeling today?

MOOD:

ENERGY:

APPETITE:

BABY MOVEMENT?

CONTRACTIONS?

If a child is to keep alive his inborn sense of wonder without any such gift from the fairies,
he needs the companionship of at least one adult who can share it, rediscovering with him the joy,
excitement and mystery of the world we live in.
RACHEL CARSON

week 30

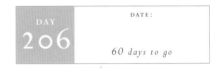

DAY 204	DATE:
	62 days to go

At this point the baby can register information from all five of its senses.

This month you may notice some increased shortness of breath. As the baby gets bigger and crowds more and more into your lungs, it's going to take more effort for you to breathe deeply. Shortness of breath does not mean oxygen deprivation for you or the baby.

Did You Know? At birth, your baby's sense of touch will be the most sensitive and well developed of all its senses.

Parenting Tips Make up your baby's crib sheets and pads in layers so all you have to do is pull off a top sheet and a pad to change the sheets.

DAY 205	DATE:
	61 days to go

While the baby's senses may be prepared to process information, certain senses have limited opportunities to operate. Since the baby doesn't breathe air inside your uterus, the sense of smell is on hold until after birth.

As the baby's due date approaches, your body is going to spend more and more time practicing for the birth. Specifically, the muscles of your uterus will practice contracting and relaxing.

Did You Know? Practice contractions are called Braxton-Hicks contractions. They are generally painless but may be experienced more frequently from now on.

Parenting Tips Set a plastic bottle of soap or lotion in the tub water with the baby so it will be warm and comfortable when you're ready to use it.

DAY 206	DATE:
	60 days to go

The colored portion, or iris, of the baby's eye is beginning to respond to the intensity of the light by opening under dim light conditions and closing under bright light conditions. This activity is automatic and is called the pupillary reflex.

Weak abdominal muscles can cause a woman to hold her shoulders too far back in order to support her uterus and keep her balance. The resulting muscle strain leads to fatigue and back pain. Keep your muscles fit by exercising regularly.

If you have any concerns about the contractions you may be experiencing—or you think you might actually be going into labor—give your practitioner a call. Don't go to the hospital or the emergency room. Ask your practitioner's advice first.

Everyone likes to think that he has done reasonably well in life, so that it comes as a shock to find our children believing differently. The temptation is to tune them out; it takes much more courage to listen.

JOHN D. ROCKEFELLER III

Parenting Tips To make baby night checks easier, put a dimmer on the light switch in the baby's room, keep a flashlight handy, or keep a few strong night-lights on. If the rail sides of the baby's crib squeak, spray nonstick vegetable spray on them or rub them with waxed paper to keep from disturbing the baby. Avoid harsher chemical lubricants because of the fumes.

DAY **207**	**DATE:** *59 days to go*

 Within the next three days, the baby's toe-nails will be fully formed.

This month you will notice many of the same symptoms you've experienced before, including backaches. The small of your back will have an increasingly difficult time balancing the load, as you and the baby get larger.

If your backache is severe and persistent, contact your practitioner.

Parenting Tips Remember to burp your baby after each feeding. Air that gets trapped in the stomach during feeding can cause discomfort and regurgita-tion. Be careful not to pat the baby too hard or you might cause it to vomit. Also, if you've given the burping a good try and you don't get anything, that's okay. If the baby seems comfortable, it's probably just fine.

DAY **208**	**DATE:** *58 days to go*

 The hair on your baby's head is growing longer. Depending on the genetic tendencies in your family and that of the baby's father, your baby will either be born with a full head of hair or a very sparse hair pattern on its scalp. Both are completely normal.

You may continue to have leg cramps, especially when you are trying to sleep.

If the soreness and pain persists, contact your practitioner so they can rule out the possibility of a blood clot in your leg.

Did You Know? The circulating hormones that are preparing your breasts for milk production also cause the mammary glands in your baby's breasts to swell. You will probably notice this temporary effect at birth. The breast tissue swelling is normal; the baby's tissues will shrink back within several days after birth.

notes

....

....

....

....

....

....

....

....

....

....

....

The thing about having a baby is that thereafter you have it.

JEAN KERR

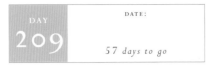

DAY
209

DATE:

57 *days to go*

By today, your baby's toenails will be fully formed.

You may notice some colostrum leaking from your breasts—it's a thin, yellowish fluid that precedes actual milk production. Colostrum will be your baby's first natural food should you decide to breast-feed. It's very nutritious and rich in antibodies.

Childbirth in Other Cultures Some new mothers in the Philippines are given a special meal after childbirth of boiled chicken, corn porridge, and a small amount of cooked placenta.

Parenting Tips Use a hand-held shower hose or even the kitchen sink sprayer when bathing a baby in a baby tub. The baby will enjoy the feel of the running water and you can wash and rinse the whole body easily—even the hair. Never let the baby hold the sprayer itself. Not only will the baby create a big mess, but it may also direct the spray into its face and risk inhaling the water.

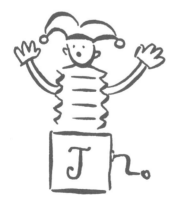

DAY
210

DATE:

56 *days to go*

Because of the rapid brain growth of the last few weeks, the circumference of your baby's head has increased by about ⅜ inch (9.5 mm). The developing brain pushes outward on the skull, but it also folds in upon itself to create more of the convolutions mentioned earlier.

Mild edema, or swelling, of your hands, feet, ankles, and face is still considered to be common, as excess fluid continues to collect in your tissues.

For Your Comfort
Drinking plenty of fluids, elevating your legs when you sit, lying on your left side, trying to maintain a comfortable body temperature, and wearing support stockings can all help you feel more comfortable.

Parenting Tips Keep cotton gloves or glove liners on your hands for a better grip when holding and washing your baby. Wet babies are slippery!

How are you feeling today?

MOOD:

ENERGY:

APPETITE:

BABY MOVEMENT?

CONTRACTIONS?

The mother-child relationship is paradoxical and, in a sense, tragic.
It requires the most intense love on the mother's side, yet this very love must help the child
grow away from the mother and to become fully independent.

ERICH FROMM

week 31

DAY	DATE:
211	*55 days to go*

As you begin Week 31, your baby is continuing to grow at an amazing rate. Right now, it measures about 11 inches long (280 mm) and weighs about 3½ pounds (1,615 g). By the time this week ends, your baby will have added almost ⅜ inch (9.5 mm) to its length.

The placenta is a very complex and complete organ. Every enzyme known to exist in biology (except ACTH) has been found in the placenta. That means the placenta can play a role in any endocrine function.

Did You Know? The word *embryo* comes from Greek words meaning "to grow in" (*en* = in and *bruein* = to grow).

Chart your waist size and weight here.

WAIST SIZE .... WEIGHT

Parenting Tips If you're bottle-feeding, prepare all the formula you'll need for the next twenty-four hours once a day, and store it in the refrigerator.

DAY	DATE:
212	*54 days to go*

Depending on its size and position in your uterus, the baby may be carried high (pressed up against your lungs) or low (pressing against your pelvis); the baby may lie in a position that makes you look wide or compact; and you may look bigger or smaller than women who are just as far along as you with their pregnancies.

You may be bothered more by constipation now than before. As your uterus becomes larger, it pushes more on your bowel, interfering with its normal activity and making it more sluggish than usual.

For Your Health Regular exercise and plenty of fruits, vegetables, juices, and fluid in your diet will be your best allies against constipation. Strong black tea is to be avoided during pregnancy because of the constipating effect of tannin.

Parenting Tips Keep two diaper pails at the dressing area: one for soiled diapers (if you use cloth diapers, fill the pail half full with water to which borax has been added so it won't get smelly) and the other for wet or soiled clothing that will later be transferred to the laundry. Use plastic bags to line the diaper pails.

What a mother sings to the cradle goes all the way down to the coffin.

HENRY WARD BEECHER

DAY 213	DATE: 53 days to go

By about this point, the volume of amniotic fluid has reached its maximum. As the baby grows, there will be less fluid and more baby and thus, you will feel considerable movement from within. The amniotic fluid is clear and straw-colored. By the time the baby is born, 2–6 cups (500–1,500 mL) of fluid fill the amniotic sac.

Your breasts will feel increasingly nodular or lumpy as they prepare for milk production. Breast changes will be most noticeable if this is your first pregnancy.

For Your Comfort
Stretching skin on your abdomen means itchy skin. Try not to scratch your itching skin even though you may be tempted to do so. Instead, apply lotion or swim to relieve skin discomfort.

Parenting Tips Save time by folding traditional cloth diapers only as you need them. Keep a laundry basket of clean, unfolded diapers near the dressing area.

DAY 214	DATE: 52 days to go

Sometimes babies at this stage practice sucking by sucking their thumbs or fingers.

Although you may be quite tired, you still may have difficulty sleeping because of backache, baby movement, feeling too hot, headaches, leg cramps, or trouble finding a comfortable position.

IMPORTANT Remember that when you lie down, try always to roll to your left side (it improves your circulation and the baby's and aids in your digestion and breathing). A full body pillow may also help achieve a comfortable position for sleeping.

Parenting Tips When bathing the baby, put a bit of cold cream or petroleum jelly on the baby's brows to channel soapy water away from its eyes.

notes

....
....
....
....
....
....
....
....
....
....
....
....
....
....

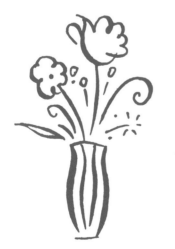

The world will never get any better until children are an improvement on their parents.
BOB EDWARDS

DAY	DATE:
215	*51 days to go*

Your baby is about 1 inch (25.4 mm) longer than it was just four days ago!

You may notice more leg fatigue and more varicose veins in your legs and abdomen. As your weight and blood volume increase, more and more pressure is placed on the veins of your legs and the legs themselves, resulting in a dull, aching pain.

For Your Comfort
Try putting on support stockings as soon as you get up in the morning to ease the achiness. Also, stay off your feet as much as possible.

Parenting Tips Use decorative kitchen canisters to hold baby items near the changing table or hang a shelf above the changing table to hold necessities and to keep items out of the reach of grasping hands when the baby becomes a toddler. A shoe bag also works well.

DAY	DATE:
216	*50 days to go*

As fat accumulates under the baby's skin, its skin color changes from dark red and transparent to pinkish (even in babies who will eventually be dark-skinned) and translucent. The baby is making its greatest demands for protein and fat now during the last half of pregnancy. In the last six to eight weeks before birth it will double its weight.

Some women are concerned about the dreams they have during pregnancy, but dreaming a lot is a normal response. When we go through transitional times in our lives—and pregnancy definitely qualifies as one—we have more worries and concerns than during the times we feel more stable. Change, even a good change like having a baby, requires adjustment, and adjustment causes stress. Worries you have during your waking hours (Will the baby be okay? Will I be a good parent? Can I handle the responsibility?) might also be examined when you dream, because they're still on your mind.

For Your Comfort
Rather than worrying uselessly, try to confront your concerns. If you're worrying about whether the baby will be healthy, take all the steps within your power to make sure you're doing the best by your pregnancy. Practice your breathing exercises during times of stress. Concentrate on breathing in slowly and steadily through your nose and then exhaling slowly and carefully from your mouth. Close your eyes and try to clear your mind of worrisome thoughts while you relax the muscles of your body. Consider meditation or prayer as a stress-control strategy.

List of parental requirements: Affection without sentiment, authority without cruelty, discipline without aggression, humor without ridicule, sacrifice without obligation, companionship without possessiveness.

WILLIAM E. BLATZ

DAY 217	DATE:
	49 days to go

At the close of this week of pregnancy, the circumference or distance around your baby's head has increased by about ⅜ inch (9.5 mm) due to its rapid brain growth.

Depending on the season of the year, it may be easier or more difficult for you to maintain a well-balanced diet. If it's winter, you might find you're hungrier, but the variety of foods isn't great. If it's summer, you may be less hungry because of the heat, but have more fresh fruits and vegetables available.

For Your Health Whatever the time of year, enjoy seasonal foods, eat several smaller meals instead of one or two larger ones, drink plenty of fluids, and take a vitamin supplement if your practitioner recommends it.

Childbirth in Other Cultures After a child's birth, the Tolong of the Philippines place the placenta in a clay pot, smoke it, and then bury the pot.

How are you feeling today?

MOOD:

ENERGY:

APPETITE:

BABY MOVEMENT?

CONTRACTIONS?

notes

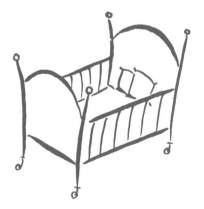

We are transfused into our children, and feel more keenly for them than for ourselves.
MARIE DE SEVEGNE

week 32

DAY	DATE:
2 1 8	48 days to go

The baby is still growing rapidly. During this week, it will grow ½ inch (13 mm) longer. From this time on, your baby has the maturity to adapt to living outside the womb if born. This is reassuring news, especially since some babies apparently can't wait to leave their cramped quarters!

Childbirth in Other Cultures In the Yucatán, massage *(sobada)* is part of each visit by the midwife. If the midwife determines that the baby is in a breech, or transverse, position, she will do an inversion, locating the baby's head and hip and applying strong, even pressure to rotate the baby's body into the more favorable head-down position. This is sometimes painful, but it is preferred over a Cesarean section.

Parenting Tips You shouldn't expect a comfortable routine to develop quickly after the birth. Adjusting to the needs and patterns of a new baby takes time, even if you've had other children. The baby's habits probably won't fit into the established routine, and expecting disruptions in the old order can make them easier to endure. Decide well before the birth who's responsible for certain chores so other family members can adapt with less confusion.

DAY	DATE:
2 1 9	47 days to go

The baby's eyes will open during the alert times of its daily cycle, and close when it sleeps. The eyes are usually blue at this time regardless of the final color they will become, because the pigmentation that colors the eye is not fully developed. Final formation of eye pigmentation generally requires a few weeks' exposure to light.

Even though your baby's eyes can now process visual information, it's difficult to imagine what the baby's world must look like to it, especially since their focusing ability is poor. Even after birth, babies usually see primary colors most clearly for a while.

Think About It
The decision about medication during labor is an individual one. Being able to "tough it out" doesn't necessarily make you more dedicated or a better mother. If, after the onset of labor, you feel you want some type of pain relief, discuss your options with your practitioner. Pain medications administered during labor do not cause birth defects.

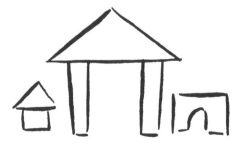

Pretty much all the honest truth telling there is in the world is done by children.
OLIVER WENDELL HOLMES

Parenting Tips Keep a prepared bag to grab as you go out of the house with your baby so you won't have to think about what to take. Keep it stocked with diapers, an extra set of clothes, wipes, a light blanket, and plastic bags (those that come in a roll are handy). Save free samples of baby products for this traveling bag and keep the containers to refill with the contents of larger size products. If bottle-feeding, keep a clean bottle set with dry formula in it; if breastfeeding, a bottle with water in it. Don't forget to restock the bag after your outing.

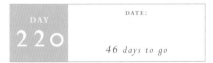

DAY 220	DATE:
	46 days to go

In addition to the immune protection provided by you, the baby is also beginning to develop its own immune reaction to mild infections.

Throughout your pregnancy, you have been supplying your baby with antibody protection to help make it immune to respiratory and gastro-intestinal infections as well as to common viral infections (like chickenpox or measles), if such antibodies are present in your system. The antibodies are passed from your bloodstream through the placenta to the baby's bloodstream.

 Talk with your practitioner about the best method of feeding your newborn.

Did You Know? If you breast-feed your baby, antibodies will continue to be passed from you to your baby and will continue to protect your child from disease. Bottle-fed babies receive no such immune protection.

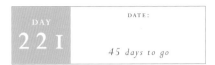

DAY 221	DATE:
	45 days to go

In the next three days, the baby's fingernails will reach the ends of the fingertips.

Most physicians don't recommend travel during the last two months of your pregnancy. Long trips by car are too exhausting; other modes of transportation place too much distance between you and your practitioner.

For Your Comfort
If you need a change of scenery, take short trips until after the baby is born.

Did You Know? At birth, the baby's umbilical cord is closed naturally by a special jellylike substance that surrounds the vessels of the cord throughout pregnancy. The jelly swells up with exposure to the air and compresses the embedded vessels like a tourniquet. Some naturally occurring hormones in the jelly also help to prevent bleeding. That's why when the cord is cut, it is practically bloodless.

notes

Each time you look at your child you see something mysterious and contradictory—bits and pieces of other people—grandparents, your mate, yourself, all captured in a certain stance, a shape of a head, a look in the eyes, combined with something very precious—a new human soul rich in individuality and possibility.

JOAN SUTTON

DAY **222**	DATE: *44 days to go*

Since the amniotic fluid volume has reached its maximum, you can now think of your baby as resting on the walls of your uterus rather than floating in fluid-filled space. It is still bathed in amniotic fluid, of course, and that fluid is replaced continuously by your efficient system.

Within the next week or so, your total blood volume will increase in anticipation of the birth. The increased blood volume adds 2–4 pounds (896–1,792 g) of weight.

Did You Know? The surface of the umbilical cord contains no pain receptors, so cutting the cord at birth is not painful for the baby or you in any way.

Parenting Tips If you breast-feed, you may find that your breasts become engorged sometimes and are quite uncomfortable. Try relieving the fullness in your breasts by expressing milk while taking a warm shower or bath if the baby isn't ready to nurse or if you're too sore to let it try. Milk flows better when you are warm. Breast pumps can also provide relief, but they don't work for everyone.

DAY **223**	DATE: *43 days to go*

By today, the baby's fingernails have reached the ends of its fingertips. You may find you have to cut its nails after birth. Even though the nails are small, they can still scratch (babies scratch themselves more often because of their poor muscle control). The newborn's face may even have some scratch marks on it from its own long fingernails.

The blood pressure in some women at this point in their pregnancy may be rather unstable. A slight drop in blood pressure can cause fainting, dizziness, and headaches.

For Your Health Change position slowly and deliberately (especially when getting up from lying prone), make sure your blood sugar doesn't drop too low (eat regularly), sit in well-ventilated areas, and try to maintain a comfortable body temperature.

Childbirth in Other Cultures In almost all cultures, both ancient and current, the placenta is wrapped up and buried after the birth.

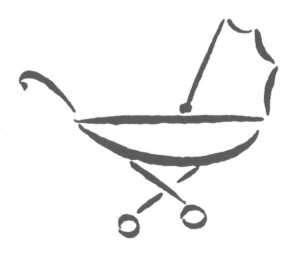

The rich don't have children; they have heirs.
PETER C. NEWMAN

DAY 224	DATE:
	42 days to go

If your baby is born now, it will not only be able to make an efficient transition from the womb to the outside, but it will also be able to resist disease.

This day marks the end of eight months (thirty-two weeks) of pregnancy. You're heading for the home stretch.

Did You Know? Your baby's growth rate is astonishing. Over the past week, its head circumference has increased by about another ⅜ inch (9.5 mm) due to its rapid brain development. The critical period for the development of the baby's brain occurs in these last months of pregnancy.

Parenting Tips If you're bottlefeeding and need to take bottled milk somewhere, pack bottles in reusable plastic ice balls or cold packs to keep the milk fresh and avoid melted ice. Place a sandwich bag or a square piece of plastic wrap across the top of the bottle before you screw on the nipples and collar ring to keep the bottle from leaking.

How are you feeling today?

Mood:

Energy:

Appetite:

Baby Movement?

Contractions?

notes

Children are poor men's riches.

ENGLISH PROVERB

Normal pregnancy lasts 9½ lunar months.

Lunar month 10 actually begins with Week 37.

Lunar Month

THINGS TO DO THIS MONTH:

Eat even if you're not especially hungry. Note that weight loss this month is common.

Be aware of fluctuating energy levels—fatigue alternating with bursts of activity.

Anticipate increased clumsiness as the baby shifts position; be aware that bumping on your
   cervix may cause light spotting.

Prevent leg cramps by resting and elevating your legs.

Prepare for birth: be sure you have provisions and clothing for the baby; begin stocking your
   freezer with easy-to-prepare foods; place a list of emergency phone numbers in a
   convenient place; and start arranging for help.

Try to stand or walk when you're having a contraction.

Urinate frequently and empty your bladder completely each time.

Continue walking for exercise and practice your breathing and relaxation exercises to reduce
   physical pain and tension.

Read books on parenting and child development.

Watch for signs of labor.

week 33

DAY 225	DATE: *41 days to go*

Right now, your baby weighs at least 4½ pounds (2,016 g) and measures about 12 inches long (300 mm).

The lunar months of pregnancy are a little deceiving. Because each lunar month has four weeks of seven days each (twenty-eight days in total), the baby actually requires 266 days, or nine and a half months, to complete development.

Childbirth in Other Cultures In what was Tanganyika in Africa and is now Tanzania, a pregnant woman's diet is enriched with meat, milk, blood, and fat.

Parenting Tips Begin childproofing the house now by moving all cleaning supplies from the spaces under sinks and cabinets and locking them in high, out-of-reach storage sites. Your baby will be crawling before you know it.

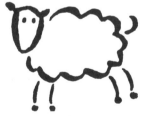

DAY 226	DATE: *40 days to go*

If the baby is a boy, his testes will have finished descending sometime between now and the due date.

Sometime within the next three days, your total blood volume will have increased from 17–21 cups (4–5½ liters) in preparation for birth. The body is anticipating some blood loss since, among other things, the placenta has to separate from the uterine wall, and it is preparing a surplus of blood so some can be lost without risk. Continue to drink plenty of fluids.

Chart your waist size and weight here.

WAIST SIZE	WEIGHT

Childbirth in Other Cultures In cultures where women play an important role in the economic structure of the society, for example, in Tierra del Fuego, women must be separated from their babies soon after childbirth so they can return to their work and responsibilities.

Parenting Tips In the summer, cover your child's car seat with a sheet, towel, or receiving blanket when not in use. The seat can become very hot and burn the baby's tender skin. Use a car shade or apply solar film to the window near the car seat.

If, in instructing a child, you are vexed with it for want of adroitness, try, if you have never tried before, to write with your left hand, and then remember that a child is all left hand.

J. F. BOYSE

DAY	DATE:
227	*39 days to go*

The baby might "drop" (shift into your pelvis) before labor begins, but not all babies drop prior to the onset of labor.

If the baby drops (this is also called "settling" or "lightening"), you will begin to notice a decrease in lap space when seated, a sudden ease of breathing and more stomach capacity (since the load has shifted down), more pelvic pressure, and more frequent urination—maybe even slight incontinence (difficulty holding your urine).

At each prenatal visit, your practitioner will check to see if the baby has dropped into your pelvis.

IMPORTANT Be aware of these pelvic sensations, but don't worry if they aren't happening according to a set schedule. While dropping or settling is expected two to four weeks before delivery, it's hard to predict the events of birth. Every baby has its own timetable.

notes

_____
_____
_____
_____
_____
_____
_____
_____
_____
_____

DAY	DATE:
228	*38 days to go*

The baby almost always settles into the mother's pelvis in a head-down position, because the head is the heaviest part of its body and is better accommodated in the bottom contour of the uterus than in the top.

Your baby will leave your uterus through the cervix (the neck, or mouth, of the uterus). When your cervix has dilated to 10 cm (4 inches), the baby can pass through.

Your practitioner will monitor your cervix for signs of dilation (widening) and effacement (thinning) at each checkup.

Did You Know? It's not uncommon for women to be dilated ⅓ to ¾ inch (1 or 2 cm) in the last month but not to be in active labor or having many noticeable contractions.

Parenting Tips Keep a baby file or baby box in which you drop an occasional note about the baby's behavior, a baby book, pictures of the baby, or, later, pictures that the baby has drawn.

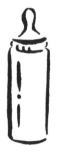

Parents are often so busy with the physical rearing of children that they miss the glory of parenthood, just as the grandeur of the trees is lost when raking leaves.

Marcelene Cox

DAY **229**	DATE: *37 days to go*

A baby delivered at eight months will tend to lose considerably more weight than a full-term baby because its digestive tract is still too immature for complete independence. As a sort of safety precaution, the eight-month fetus stores nutrition from its mother against the possibility of an early birth.

Between weeks 16 and 40, 15–20% more oxygen is captured by your lungs from each volume of air you breathe.

Your practitioner will probably want to see you once a week until you go into labor. Make sure you keep your appointments, since it's important to monitor the frequency and duration of your contractions (if you have any), to determine if the baby has dropped, to assess swelling, weight gain, and blood pressure, and to test for protein and sugar in the urine.

Parenting Tips When you visit your practitioner, take written notes of any verbal instructions they give you. What seems clear in the office may become confusing by the time you get home. Bring a list of questions with you so you won't forget to ask. Never be afraid to ask a question about anything that pertains to you or your baby.

DAY **230**	DATE: *36 days to go*

The pinkness of the baby's skin (both now and at birth) is due to blood vessels that are close to the surface. Even babies who will have dark skin later on have skin with a pinkish cast now.

Your diaphragm is now elevated and tilted because of pressure from your enlarging uterus. This change causes your rib cage to flair, or open up slightly. The circumference of your chest may increase by almost 2½ inches (61mm).

IMPORTANT You may notice stronger and more frequent Braxton-Hicks contractions, some of which may even be painful. This is normal.

Parenting Tips When parents aren't around, babies soothe themselves with what are known as transitional objects—physical comforts that help ease a child's fear of separating from caregivers. For that reason, consider fostering such attachments early in your child's infancy by offering it a special blanket, plush toy, or a pacifier. A child's reliance on a transitional object is not a sign of insecurity—it's a coping mechanism.

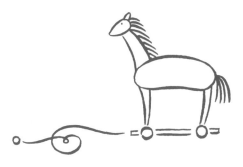

A small boy, mischievous to the imp degree.
REA MURTHA

DAY **2 3 1**	**DATE:** *35 days to go*

The baby's arms and legs are beginning to be chubby as more fat is deposited. Fat deposits increase from about 2% at midpregnancy to 12–15% at term.

Iron transfer takes place at the placenta in one direction only: from you toward the baby. Five-sixths of the iron stored in the baby's liver accumulates during the last trimester. The stored iron will compensate in the baby's first four months out of the womb for inadequate amounts of iron in breast milk or formulas, so make sure your iron intake is adequate.

For Your Comfort
During this last month, give yourself more opportunity to rest and relax. Elevate your legs when you can and drink plenty of fluids.

Parenting Tips You might not think infants really care which toys you choose to give them, as long as they're soft, cuddly, or make a funny noise; however, some toys can support the development of the child's early skills. For example, first toys might include those that are visually stimulating since the baby's eyes are learning to process form, line, shape, and color. Mobiles and high-contrast visual displays are good choices.

notes

How are you feeling today?

MOOD:

ENERGY:

APPETITE:

BABY MOVEMENT?

CONTRACTIONS?

Children don't have to be raised. They'll grow.
BUFFY SAINTE-MARIE

week 34

DAY **232**	DATE:
	34 days to go

The baby has developed for thirty-three weeks. Receiving nutrition and elimination through the umbilical cord all this time has made it unnecessary for the baby's slowly developing gastrointestinal system to function much before birth. Even after birth, this system will still be physiologically immature until the child is three or four years old.

Your basal metabolism rate increases 25% late in your pregnancy, so your body is now 25% more efficient in converting stored nutrients to energy. This increase is in response to the continuing demands of the baby on your system and the needs of your body's tissues.

Did You Know? From this point on, the "finishing period" of growth begins, during which your baby prepares for its birth.

Parenting Tips To avoid your baby crying when you leave it with others, try spending a few minutes with the child before leaving and not rushing off hurriedly.

DAY **233**	DATE:
	33 days to go

During this finishing period of the baby's development, fat is being laid down under the surface of the baby's skin, which will help the baby maintain an even body temperature and which can be burned as energy. Growth has slowed—perhaps to conserve energy for the birth process.

A diet providing 2,400 calories is generally recommended at this point in your pregnancy to meet your energy requirements—unless you are physically inactive.

Did You Know? You may actually begin to lose weight this month. Weight loss of 2–3 pounds (896–1,344g) is not uncommon as labor approaches and the baby's development is completed.

IMPORTANT Never leave a baby alone, except in its crib, playpen, or other secure place. Always pick up the baby and take it with you when you answer the phone or door, even if that means taking it out of the bathwater to do so. It only takes a second for an unsupervised baby to get into serious trouble.

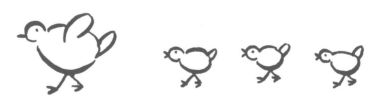

No animal is so inexhaustible as an excited infant.

AMY LESLIE

DAY	DATE:
234	*32 days to go*

The baby's limbs are beginning to dimple at the elbows and knees, and creases are forming around the wrists and neck as fat deposit continues.

The circulatory requirements of your uterus have increased throughout your pregnancy as it enlarged and the baby and placenta developed. Now, near the end of your pregnancy, one-sixth of your total blood volume is contained within the vessels of the uterus.

IMPORTANT You'll notice more fluctuations in your energy level this month. Fatigue is experienced by most pregnant women, but this month, you may find that fatigue alternates with periods of extra energy. Use your energy bursts wisely doing things you absolutely need to do and preparing for the birth and time after birth. Don't overdo it, though! You might need to conserve some of that energy for later.

Parenting Tips Before your baby begins to crawl, cover all unused electrical outlets with pronged plastic caps, available at hardware stores. Wind up excess lengths of plugged-in cords and fasten with rubber bands or twist ties.

DAY	DATE:
235	*31 days to go*

The baby's gums are now ridged and may look at first like teeth are about to erupt.

During labor, the amniotic fluid that surrounds the baby equalizes the pressure of the contractions, so one part of the baby's body is not pressed more than another. The amniotic fluid also prevents contractions from interfering with the blood flow from the placenta to the baby.

IMPORTANT Your baby needs to eat even when you'd rather not. Several small meals a day are still best at this point for most women.

Parenting Tips Devise different names to call grandparents so your child can learn to tell them apart when people are speaking about them. Some grandparents choose their own names (Grandpa Joe or Grandma Jones) and some prefer nicknames.

notes

Call it a clan, call it a network, call it a tribe, call it a family.
Whatever you call it, whoever you are, you need one.

JANE HOWARD

DAY 236	DATE:
	30 days to go

By the time the baby is born, the placenta will weigh one-sixth of what the baby weighs. While your appetite and energy levels might fluctuate, you'll probably notice more rather than less swelling of your ankles, feet, hands, and face during these final weeks. About 40% of women have slight ankle swelling during the last twelve weeks of pregnancy. This swelling generally disappears with rest and is rarely present in the morning.

Any swelling you have that is associated with pain or swelling that does not disappear within twenty-four hours should be reported to your practitioner.

For Your Information Clear-or pink-tinged mucous may be a sign that the mucous plug, which seals the opening of the uterus, has dislodged. This usually means that the cervix is beginning to dilate and that true labor may be days or even hours away.

IMPORTANT Don't place the baby's crib or other furniture near a window. If the window is open, the child might fall out.

notes

DAY 237	DATE:
	29 days to go

Within the next day or so, the percentage of white fat in the baby's body will have increased to 8%.

As your growing uterus puts pressure on your diaphragm, your heart will become displaced upward and to the left.

For Your Comfort
Leg cramps during sleep are common late in pregnancy. Prevent cramps by avoiding fatigue and elevating your legs whenever possible.

Parenting Tips Cut your infant's nails at a time when they are distracted and you have both hands free. A good time might be when the baby is nursing or asleep or when their head is propped on a pillow so you don't have to support them in place. Use nail clippers or round-end scissors for speed and safety.

A child's education should begin at least one hundred years before he is born.
OLIVER WENDELL HOLMES

DAY 238

DATE:

28 days to go

It took eight weeks for the baby's body fat percentage to increase from 2–3% (Week 26) to 8% (Week 34). By the end of prenatal development, the baby's body fat percentage will stabilize at about 15%. This protective padding of fat will keep the baby warm after birth.

Your baby may become quite chubby if you overeat during this time. Even with normal weight gain, the baby now fits snugly in your womb and can only turn from side to side.

Childbirth in Other Cultures In some cultures such as China, breast-feeding continues for up to six years.

Parenting Tips A good diet, good hygiene, and regular checkups are essential to your baby's dental health. Consider cleaning your infant's first teeth with a small gauze pad, with or without toothpaste. Place the child on your lap with its head by your knees and rub the pad over the teeth and gums very gently to remove plaque and leftover food.

How are you feeling today?

MOOD:

ENERGY:

APPETITE:

BABY MOVEMENT?

CONTRACTIONS?

notes

No one has yet fully realized the wealth of sympathy, kindness and generosity hidden in the soul of a child. The effort of every true education should be to unlock that treasure.

EMMA GOLDMAN

week 35

DAY	DATE:
239	27 days to go

Eighty-five percent of babies are born within two weeks of their due dates, either early or late. You and the baby have entered that time frame now.

Your vaginal discharge will become heavier now and will contain more cervical mucous. The discharge may be streaked with recent (reddish or pink) or oxidized (brown) blood after intercourse or after a pelvic exam.

IMPORTANT Watch for symptoms of labor, but don't be obsessed with them. Your baby's birthday could be just around the corner or it could be weeks away. Take it one day at a time.

Did You Know? Your cervix is sensitive and blood-engorged right now; bumping or manipulating it may cause spotting.

Chart your waist size and weight here.

WAIST SIZE _____ WEIGHT _____

DAY	DATE:
240	26 days to go

The baby's grasp is becoming firmer and firmer.

Fetal blood flows through two umbilical arteries and one umbilical vein. During late pregnancy, a soft blowing sound called "funic souffle" can be heard over the location of your baby's umbilical cord.

Bright red discharge or persistent spotting should be reported to your practitioner immediately.

Parenting Tips

If your baby needs to take liquid medicine, give the medicine in a nipple. Flush the nipple afterward with a little water for the child to suck to make sure all the medicine is taken. A medicine dropper is also helpful. Squirt the medicine into the cheek area, not down the throat, to avoid a mess.

notes

The best inheritance a parent can give his children is a few minutes of his time each day.

O. A. Battista

DAY	DATE:
241	*25 days to go*

While the ossification process has been progressing steadily (cartilage turning into bone), not all of the baby's bones will be ossified by birth. This is an advantage for both of you. The baby's skeleton is more flexible when it contains more cartilage, making the passage through the narrow birth canal easier. Fewer hard bones means fewer hard pokes during delivery.

The total weight of the placenta and supporting membranes at term is 1½ pounds (672 g). The total weight of the amniotic fluid at term is 2 pounds (896 g).

Take Note The mucous plug, which seals the opening of the uterus, is often mistaken for amniotic fluid. The key difference is that the mucous plug is thick and looks like clear nasal mucous or mucous tinged with blood, while amniotic fluid is watery.

Parenting Tips Always set a timer when you're cooking with children around. Babies are distracting, and you can easily forget your food and cause a fire or ruin the food.

notes

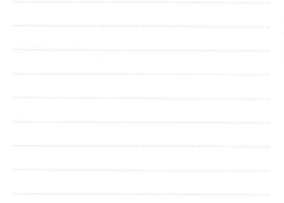

DAY	DATE:
242	*24 days to go*

The baby will now automatically turn toward a source of light. This is called the "orienting response" and permits the baby to practice being more aware of its environment.

There is generally no physiological rise in blood pressure during a healthy pregnancy, in spite of the increased blood volume and increased demands on your heart. In fact, your blood pressure may have been slightly lower than normal during the second trimester. It will be highest during the last week of your pregnancy.

IMPORTANT Basically, your baby will need clothing, diapers, a place to sleep, food, and love after birth. You can supply the love and the food (if you're breast-feeding), but do you have everything else you'll need for the first couple of weeks after delivery?

Parenting Tips Many young infants become extremely distressed when they are undressed. They hate the feeling of air on their bodies and prefer to be fully clothed or tucked snugly into their blankets. When the baby is very young, you can give it a sponge bath, washing its face and around its ears with a damp cotton ball or a wash cloth, while keeping its undershirt and diaper in place. If you need to change the baby's shirt, make sure its diaper or pajama bottoms are still on.

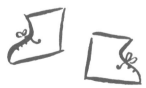

Babies: Little rivets in the bonds of matrimony.
ARTHUR GORDON

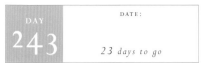

DAY 243

DATE:

23 days to go

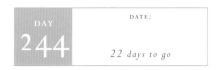

DAY 244

DATE:

22 days to go

The baby's body is taking on a rounded, fuller look as the weight it gains is primarily white, subcutaneous body fat.

Braxton-Hicks contractions—false labor pains—are believed to facilitate circulation to and through the placenta by stimulating the movement of the blood.

For Your Comfort
It's important to plan ahead, so you can relax as much as possible before and during delivery, knowing everything has been taken care of. If you have a freezer, you and your partner might begin stocking it with easy-to-prepare foods.

Parenting Tips If you use cloth diapers, you can use diaper wraps, diaper clips (like tiny clamps), or conventional diaper pins to keep diapers snug. If you use pins, be sure you select the ones with covered plastic ends, because they're less likely to come unfastened and poke the baby. Stick pins in a bar of soap with the wrapping left on or in a decorative candle to help them slide through the cloth easier. Never hold diaper pins in your mouth—babies are great imitators.

The baby maintains a temperature of about 32°F above maternal temperature.

Because the baby's quarters are so cramped at this point, when it moves, the contours of its arms and legs make moving bulges on your abdomen. It should be fairly easy for you to identify the baby's arms and legs, but you may confuse the head with the buttocks through the stretched skin of your abdomen.

Did You Know? You will notice that for several weeks after birth, your baby will maintain the fetal position it was forced to assume in the uterus, because its muscles are used to it.

IMPORTANT Everybody needs help with a new baby. Start arranging for that help now. For example, perhaps a friend could help by bringing lunch by for several days after the birth. If the people you know are inclined to give gifts, perhaps you could suggest they give the gift of assistance (bringing over nutritious meals, staying with the baby in the afternoon so you can take a nap, cleaning up a bit, etc.). On the other hand, you may be too tired for company!

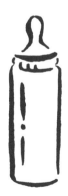

Children are the wisdom of the nation.
LIBERIAN PROVERB

DAY	DATE:
245	*21 days to go*

 This date ends Week 35 of the baby's development. From this point forward the baby's growth will be much slower until birth, except for fat production.

As you approach delivery, the amniotic sac (bag of waters) may break. Generally, it's more of a trickle than a gush. If you're concerned about fluid leakage when you're not at home, wear a pad or panty liner to absorb the moisture. Amniotic fluid has its own distinct odor and can easily be distinguished from urine.

Contact your practitioner if you think you're leaking amniotic fluid.

Parenting Tips Keep a cardboard box in each closet. As clothes are outgrown or no longer worn, place them in the bag. When the time comes for a garage sale or donation, the sorting will already be done. Unless, of course, you plan to have more children.

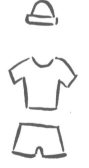

notes

How are you feeling today?

MOOD:

ENERGY:

APPETITE:

BABY MOVEMENT?

CONTRACTIONS?

You have to ask children and birds how cherries and strawberries taste.

J. W. GOETHE

week 36

DAY	DATE:
246	*20 days to go*

The baby's intestines are accumulating considerable meconium, a dark-green mass of cells and waste product from the baby's liver, pancreas, and gall bladder.

You've probably discussed the difference between false labor and true labor with your practitioner. The main points will be reviewed over the next several journal days to keep them fresh in your mind.

FALSE vs. TRUE LABOR: With Braxton-Hicks, or false labor, contractions, the pain begins in your lower abdomen. The contractions that accompany true labor begin in your lower back and the pain spreads to your lower abdomen.

Childbirth in Other Cultures In the Yucatán Peninsula, usually only the midwife, husband, and pregnant woman's mother are present at a birth. If the labor is long and difficult, other women will appear: mother-in-law, sisters, godmother, sisters-in-law, close friends, and neighbors.

Parenting Tips Apply cold for bumps and bruises in the first twenty-four hours after the injury by pressing lightly for 20 minutes. Frozen Popsicles can be useful in treating bumped lips; a bag of frozen vegetables works well as a flexible compress. A can of frozen fruit juice is a good, nondrippy compress.

DAY	DATE:
247	*19 days to go*

The meconium in the baby's intestines will be eliminated shortly after birth, but it sometimes can be eliminated before, if the birth is delayed too long. In the latter case, fecal material will be present at birth in the amniotic fluid.

By today, the baby's toenails have reached the end of the toes. After the baby is born, you may need to trim its fingernails and toenails.

If you feel like you have extra energy, save it for your labor—don't weed your entire garden or strip and wax your floors!

Parenting Tips Never leave plastic bags where children can find them. Even small pieces of plastic can cause children to suffocate. Get in the habit of knotting all plastic bags before throwing them away.

notes

We have here a baby. It is composed of a bald head and a pair of lungs.
EUGENE FIELD

DAY **248**	DATE: *18 days to go*

Within the next three days, the circumference of the baby's head will roughly match the circumference of its shoulders and its hips.

FALSE vs. TRUE LABOR: The contractions of true labor become progressively stronger and more painful as time passes and aren't interrupted by changing one's position.

Childbirth in Other Cultures In the Mayan culture, a midwife gives a woman a special massage twenty days after she gives birth. This massage marks the end of the postpartum period.

Parenting Tips If the baby isn't feeling well and you want to take its temperature, a rectal thermometer is the most accurate. The rectal thermometer will insert easier if you put petroleum jelly on it first. An ear thermometer can also be used. If you don't want to use a thermometer, there are heat-sensitive strips that one places on the baby's forehead. You can also tell if the baby is warm by pressing your lips to its forehead—the temperature of your lips is more stable than that of your hands. Be sure to tell your practitioner which method you used when you report a temperature.

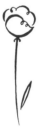

DAY **249**	DATE: *17 days to go*

As you might expect, the baby's limbs are bent and drawn close to its body. Because of the space limitations in the uterus now, the movements of the baby are quite restricted.

FALSE vs. TRUE LABOR: When timing contractions (your practitioner will have you look for contractions a certain number of minutes apart), don't expect perfect, even intervals (i.e., contraction, 6 minutes/3 seconds, contraction, 6 minutes/3 seconds, etc.). If, for example, you are supposed to call your practitioner when your contractions are four minutes apart, expect them to be about four minutes apart rather than exactly four minutes apart.

Childbirth in Other Cultures In the old times, when a Comanche Indian woman went into labor, she would go to a clearing a short distance from her camp where three four-foot stakes were set in the ground ten feet apart. She would walk while she labored, and during each contraction, would kneel down near a stake and grasp it on a level with her head. She was assisted by a female relative.

Parenting Tips When you pick your newborn up, be sure to place one hand under the baby's neck to support its head and the other hand under its back and bottom to support its lower half. Head support is particularly important—the baby will have no control over it at all until it's about four weeks old.

Parents: People who spend half their time wondering how their children will turn out, and the rest of the time when they will turn in.

Eleanor Graham Vance

DAY 250	DATE:
	16 days to go

By today, the circumference of the baby's head and abdomen are about equal.

FALSE vs. TRUE LABOR: If you stand or walk when you're having a contraction, the force of gravity will make the contractions more efficient and will reduce the time of labor. By the end of pregnancy, the smooth muscle cells of the vagina are enlarged and the supportive connective tissues are reduced. Thus, the vaginal walls have become sufficiently relaxed to permit the passage of the baby during birth.

Childbirth in Other Cultures Among the Santa Maria Indians of Guatemala, it is the custom for the midwife, both grandmothers, the husband, and sometimes the father-in-law to attend birth.

Parenting Tips Baby wipes are versatile! You can also use them to (1) clean scrapes and bruises, (2) remove eye makeup, (3) clean hands after pumping gas, (4) soothe sunburn, (5) wipe down bathroom surfaces, and (6) substitute for toilet paper for your toilet-training toddler.

DAY 251	DATE:
	15 days to go

If your baby is a girl, over the last three or so days the labia majora has formed over the labia minora.

Frequent urination can help labor progress: a full bladder will push against the uterus, causing discomfort.

Childbirth in Other Cultures A Mayan woman who sits behind the laboring mother and supports her arms and body is called the "head helper." She supports the mother's weight and shadows the mother's pushing and breathing during contractions.

Parenting Tips When you're out of the house with the baby, you might want to use a fanny pack or belt pack to hold your wallet, checkbook, and other necessities so you'll have one less thing to carry.

notes

....
....
....
....
....
....
....
....
....
....
....

Every baby born into the world is a finer one than the last.
CHARLES DICKENS

DAY 252	DATE:
	14 days to go

At this point in development, the average baby weighs about 6 pounds (2778 g) and measures about 13 ⅜ inches (340 mm).

Use relaxation exercises such as deep breathing to help ease the pain of the contractions.

Childbirth in Other Cultures A number of tribes lubricate a laboring woman's birth canal with saps or oils to make the delivery easier.

Parenting Tips It's common for babies to develop a fear of shampooing, as soap and water sometimes makes its way into little eyes. To avoid these problems, place colorful stickers on the ceiling over the tub to get the baby to look up—then you can rinse the suds off. Use a sponge instead of a cup to control the flow of water.

How are you feeling today?

Mood:

Energy:

Appetite:

Baby Movement?

Contractions?

notes

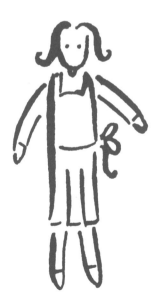

Once you bring life into this world, you must protect it. We must protect it by changing the world.

Elie Weisel

week 37

Contrary to popular understanding, human gestation actually requires nine and a half lunar months, not nine. These last two weeks are for that additional period. Over the next few days, the baby's skin will become thicker and paler.

FALSE vs. TRUE LABOR: The contractions of true labor may be accompanied by diarrhea.

Childbirth in Other Cultures If a laboring woman is tiring or progress is slowing, many cultures know to stimulate the woman's nipples so that oxytocin will be released into her system. This is the same substance that is used in synthetic form in the United States and other Western cultures to induce labor.

Parenting Tips Diaper rash is something that almost all babies experience. Changing diapers frequently can help avoid it. If a rash does develop, expose the baby's bottom to the air when it naps (the bedding can be protected by folding a towel under the baby as it sleeps) or let the baby stay bare-bottomed at times when awake. Drying the baby's bottom between diaper changes with a hand-held hairdryer helps, too (use a "warm," not "hot," setting and hold well away from the skin to avoid burning). Don't use baby wipes premoistened with alcohol, as they can be too drying.

Over the next couple of days, the baby's lungs will begin to increase their production of a surfactant, which will keep the air sacs in the lungs open.

Your uterus is highly muscular and weighs 2½ pounds (1,120 g) now that the baby is fully developed. During a contraction, the uterus feels hard to the touch.

Chart your waist size and weight here.

WAIST SIZE .... WEIGHT ....

IMPORTANT Be prepared to call your practitioner when signs indicate that you're ready to go to the hospital or birth center or to begin the process of home birth. Don't worry about the time of day. People who attend births expect to be called at all hours!

Parenting Tips Some parents keep a notebook for each child, recording all medical, legal, and school information. Alternatively, file cards can be used to list illnesses, dates of vaccinations, teachers in school, etc.

Boy: A noise with some dirt on it.
SAMUEL TAYLOR COLERIDGE

DAY	DATE:
255	*11 days to go*

From about this point on, the baby will gain about ½ ounce (14 g) of fat each day it stays in your uterus.

The muscles at the top of your uterus apply a force comparable to a weight of 55 pounds (24.6 kg) during each contraction. This shows how much force must be applied to resistant muscles to open the cervix and push the baby out of the uterus during birth.

IMPORTANT Keep your list of emergency phone numbers in a convenient place. If you're in labor and can't get to the hospital or in touch with your midwife, dial 911 or the emergency number for your area. Unlock your door, lie down, and pant to avoid pushing until help arrives. Labor can take many hours, however, so don't panic if you must wait a little while for a ride.

Parenting Tips Make sure your children will be well cared for while you are giving birth. Even if you will be at home, you can't attend to their needs during labor and delivery (even for a while afterward). Arrange for someone to be there to watch your children.

DAY	DATE:
256	*10 days to go*

The lanugo (downy hair that once covered the baby's body) is disappearing. If any of the lanugo remains by birth, it will be found on the baby's shoulders, forehead, and neck.

FALSE vs. TRUE LABOR: You might be interested in other women's descriptions of the experience of true labor. Many women compare the contractions of true labor to waves: gathering, rising, breaking, falling. The pressure builds in the uterine muscles and reaches a peak that lasts thirty to fifty seconds or so. Then the pressure disappears rapidly. When it's over you feel nothing until the next contraction. To some, the gripping sensation of the contraction feels like bad menstrual cramps or intestinal cramps. Most women report that persistent backache accompanies the contractions. Labor is a well-named phenomenon. It's the work that you will do to bear your baby. Although the work is difficult, few jobs are as rewarding or satisfying.

Childbirth in Other Cultures Many cultures believe that the placenta needs to be treated in a special way because it is part of the baby's soul.

For Your Comfort
Citrus drops or herbal throat drops are nice to have on hand during labor to help keep your mouth from drying.

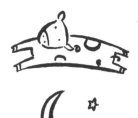

The toughest thing about raising kids is convincing them that you have seniority.
ANONYMOUS

DAY 257	DATE:
	9 days to go

Your newborn will have no functioning tear ducts for a couple of weeks. The first cries are always tearless ones.

There are many reasons why you might have more difficulty sleeping from now on. The baby may be much more active, you may be experiencing periodic contractions, and you're probably anxious and anticipating the birth. All of this is very predictable and common.

IMPORTANT Try to relax and be as comfortable as you can. Rest whenever you feel tired.

Parenting Tips Some parents might want to involve existing siblings in the birth event. Homebirth and birthing centers can accommodate children. The age and personality of each individual child is an important consideration. Not all children will react positively to childbirth. Some children might be fascinated by all the activity; some might be scared; some might be bored and restless. Make sure you have someone on hand to take care of the needs of the attending children. If the siblings are hungry or tired or want to do something else, this caretaking adult can take over and see that their needs are met in a safe and timely way.

DAY 258	DATE:
	8 days to go

The average length of a newborn's umbilical cord is 2 feet (610 mm), but the cord can vary from 5 inches (127 mm) to more than 4 feet (1219 mm) long. By the time of birth, the cord is capable of carrying about 300 quarts (302.3 L) of fluid per day.

When the baby settles deep into your pelvis, you may feel clumsy and off-balance. That's because your center of gravity has shifted as the baby changed its position.

Childbirth in Other Cultures In many tribal cultures, a mother and newborn baby stay in their own hut, where they rest and recuperate without distraction, away from the other members of their group.

Parenting Tips A video camera is an expensive, but invaluable investment. Consider dedicating one cassette each to Birthdays, Holidays, Visits with Relatives, etc. so that, cumulative video records will be kept of the child's special events from year to year. Later on, such tapes make for wonderful viewing for the child and the rest of the family.

notes

....

....

....

....

....

....

Hit a child and quarrel with its mother.

NIGERIAN PROVERB

DAY 259

DATE:

7 days to go

The color of the baby's skin is beginning to change from reddish or pinkish to white or bluish pink (even in babies with dark pigmentation). Changes in the baby's skin color are due to the growing thickness of the fatty layer under the skin's surface. Earlier in development, the skin was so transparent and the body contained so little subcutaneous fat that if you could have seen the baby, you would have seen its organs through its skin. Now, the growing layer of fat gives the baby's skin an opaque quality and masks the color of the muscles and circulating blood cells.

Week 37 draws to a close. You may notice more of a change in your gait, since your balance is being thrown off by your enlarged uterus and the shifting position of the baby.

Childbirth in Other Cultures Tribal societies tend to have a fairly long transition period after birth, during which the baby is nursed and cared for by the mother, sleeps with the mother, and is attended to quickly when it cries. The more industrialized a society is, the shorter the transition period. Scandinavian countries, like Sweden and Denmark, are the exception. They offer generous parental leaves to their citizens.

Parenting Tips During its first year, take a picture of your baby each month at about the same time (first week, third week, on the 15th, etc.). If the picture is taken in the same pose or by the same furniture, it will be easier to see the dramatic changes in the baby's growth. After the first year, take photo records at least twice a year.

How are you feeling today?

MOOD:

ENERGY:

APPETITE:

BABY MOVEMENT?

CONTRACTIONS?

notes

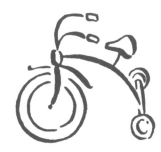

We've had bad luck with our kids—they've all grown up.
CHRISTOPHER MORLEY

week 38

DAY 260	DATE:
	6 days to go

The baby's skull is not yet fully solid. It is made up of five large bony plates that are still separated and can be pushed together, which they will be during birth.

During these last few weeks in the womb, the baby continues to receive one of the most important ingredients for survival from your blood, from the placenta, and also from the amniotic fluid (which is swallowed periodically): disease-combating antibodies that will provide an immunity to a wide range of diseases.

For Your Health Don't push yourself right now. Just rest, eat well, and nurture yourself as the baby's due date approaches.

Parenting Tips If you're away from the house and have to change diapers, place a blanket in your open trunk and change the baby there. If you have a station wagon, change the baby on the open tailgate. Both of these alternatives avoid crouching uncomfortably in the back seat of a car. Be careful of oil and gasoline residue and any sharp corners.

DAY 261	DATE:
	5 days to go

Over the next three days, the last of the vernix will begin to disappear. The sutures or spaces between the bony plates of the baby's skull are also called fontanels, which means "little fountains" because the pulse of the baby's bloodstream can be easily felt by touching them. The best known of the fontanels is the "soft spot" on the top of the baby's head. Don't worry if the baby's head becomes molded or elongated during the birth process. It will return to its normal, rounded shape a few days after childbirth. The molding is a safety precaution—the bones of the skull carefully slide over one another to reduce the skull's diameter, so the pressure of birth doesn't damage the baby's brain.

Most babies drop into a head first, face down position in their mother's pelvis. In some cases, the baby is in a head first, face up position, so the back of its head presses against the mother's tailbone or spine. This produces the phenomenon called "back labor." The pain of back labor is especially intense and doesn't seem to let up, even between contractions. Consult with your practitioner about techniques to relieve the pain.

For Your Health From now until the baby is born, continue walking for exercise and practice your breathing and relaxation exercises. If your back is particularly sore, you might try to relieve some of the pain by gently stretching those muscles. When you begin having contractions, walking and controlled breathing will both help you through them.

Happy is he that is happy in his children.

THOMAS FULLER

Parenting Tips If you have to travel by plane, carry a small infant in a front pack so you can have your arms free. Nurse your baby or give it a bottle or a pacifier during takeoff and landing to reduce the pressure in its ears.

DAY **262**	DATE: _____ *4 days to go*

Over the next three days, the baby's chest will become more prominent. The baby's abdomen will be big and round at birth because of the size of the liver. The baby's liver will be naturally large because of the special role it has had in the production of blood cells.

A kick from the womb during this stage of pregnancy can almost knock a book off your lap!

For Your Comfort
If holidays or other celebrations that you actively plan or participate in are approaching, shift responsibilities to other family members or friends for right now. You need to have all pressures taken off so you can concentrate on the birth of your baby.

Parenting Tips Your baby has gotten used to feeling snug and secure in your uterus and, after birth, may sleep better and feel more comfortable if the pre-birth environment is duplicated. Try bundling the baby gently in a receiving blanket. Place it on its side so it can feel the mattress with its face. Back placement is also advised if the head end of the mattress is elevated slightly.

notes

It is the fortune commonly of knavish children to have the lovings't mothers.
THOMAS MIDDLETON

DAY 263	DATE:
	3 days to go

If any of the vernix (the creamy protective substance on the surface of the baby's skin) remains until birth, it is usually found only on the baby's back. As the vernix sloughs off the baby's skin, the amniotic fluid may change from clear and straw-colored to milky.

If you took a childbirth preparation class, you know how useful the information you received has been. Now is a good time to review your notes.

Parenting Tips At this point, you might consider taking a parenting class or doing some reading on child development.

Childbirth in Other Cultures In Burma, new mothers are traditionally fed a soup made with fish, plants, and fruit.

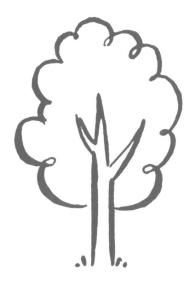

DAY 264	DATE:
	2 days to go

The first breaths the baby takes are the hardest. It has been calculated that the first breathing-in requires five times the effort of an ordinary breath, because the air drawn in must expand the thousands of tiny uninflated air sacs of the lungs. It is an effort that can be compared to blowing up a balloon.

If you're planning to breastfeed, you are going to be offering the most well-balanced, immune-protective nutrition available to your baby. Each of your breasts gains 1½ pounds (672 g) during pregnancy in preparation for nursing.

Did You Know? Because breast-feeding is a learned skill and not an instinct, make sure you have lined up support from experienced nursing mothers. You may need to call on them for advice or encouragement after the baby is born.

Parenting Tips When the baby was in your uterus, its world sounded watery and sloshy. While you can go out and buy a toy that duplicates intrauterine sounds, the sound of running water is also soothing to the baby and will help lull it to sleep. Tape-record the sound of a running shower, water filling the tub, or a running dishwasher—or buy a recording of water sounds—and play it if your baby is having trouble falling asleep.

Pretty much all the honest truth telling there is in the world is done by children.
OLIVER WENDELL HOLMES

DAY **265**	DATE:
	1 day to go

By this time, about 15% of the baby's body is fat. About 80% of this fat is located directly under the surface of the baby's skin, while the other 20% is found on organs and muscle tissue.

Your weight gain has probably slowed or even reversed itself in the past two weeks or so.

IMPORTANT Be careful when using a microwave to warm milk or food for your baby. Microwaving heats formula unevenly and creates hotspots that can scald the baby's mouth. If you express and freeze breastmilk, let it thaw by setting it in a pan of warm water. Breastmilk is the only milk that provides the baby with immune protection, and these immune bodies are destroyed by microwaving.

How are you feeling today?

MOOD: ....

ENERGY: ....

APPETITE: ....

BABY MOVEMENT? ....

CONTRACTIONS? ....

DAY **266**	DATE:
	Due date

Today is the baby's estimated due date. The baby is considered full-term at this point. That means that all of the development that takes place before birth has been accomplished. If born today, your baby will weigh about 7⅓ pounds (3,285 g) and will measure at least 15 inches (381 mm) in length.

As you get to this point, you will find that you have more and more trouble sleeping and getting around. It's difficult to find any comfortable position, and if the baby is moving frequently or if you are experiencing Braxton-Hicks contractions, you may not be able to sleep even when you are comfortable. Try to relax and rest when you can. It's difficult to be on any type of routine now.

Chart your waist size and weight here.

WAIST SIZE	WEIGHT

Childbirth in Other Cultures In cultures where new mothers spend more solitary time with their babies, births tend to be spaced fairly far apart. In cultures where women are given less transition time after the birth and return to work and household chores sooner, births tend to be more closely spaced.

Parenting Tips Eliminate all air from bottles with disposable liners by rolling up the liner from the bottom until the liquid reaches the tip of the nipples. With all the air removed, the baby will be able to drink in an upright position.

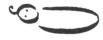

We can't give our children the future, strive though we may to make it secure. But we can give them the present.
KATHLEEN NORRIS

Full Term Plus 1

If your baby's due date came and went, don't worry—you're not going to be pregnant forever. Remember that the due date was just an estimate, and while the baby's prenatal development has been completed, every baby is different and will be born in its own time.

Full Term Plus 2

Scientists are still not exactly sure what triggers the process of labor. It might involve the weight and size of the fetus putting pressure on the cervix, as well as the biochemical balance of your body—especially since the uterus becomes more and more sensitive to certain enzymes and hormones as pregnancy continues. Walking sometimes encourages the onset of labor. Remember not to walk too fast or too far. Even if it doesn't trigger labor, walking is still good exercise.

Full Term Plus 3

If you're feeling a little impatient to give birth, that's okay. It's normal to want to get on with the process, even though you know it will be difficult and somewhat painful. Sometimes, however, impatience leads to feeling anxious and upset. It's important to stay as calm and composed as you can. Emotional distress is not going to be productive; in fact, it's going to tax your energy reserves. Try to distract yourself away from negative emotions if you can't be positive and hopeful. Just hold on. You can do it.

Full Term Plus 4

So what's going on now that you and your baby are in this holding pattern? The baby is quite prepared for life outside the womb. Its lungs are still manufacturing large quantities of surfactant, in order to keep the air sacs of the lungs open. In general, the baby just continues to grow. Its hair gets longer, the nails grow, it puts on more weight. If the baby is growing so large that a vaginal birth would be difficult, your practitioner may suggest that your labor be induced or a Cesarean section performed.

Full Term Plus 5

Your body literally can't be pregnant forever. The placenta is an extremely functional organ, but it's disposable. It can sustain a normal human pregnancy, but begins to break down in the weeks that follow the due date. Your practitioner will monitor placental functioning. Helping the placenta stay healthy involves the same activities on your part as keeping the developing baby healthy.

. . . all the time we wondered and wondered
who is this person coming / growing / turning / floating / swimming deep, deep inside.

CRESCENT DRAGONWAGON

Full Term Plus 6

While humans don't have the shortest pregnancies compared to other species, we certainly don't have the longest either. The Asiatic elephant (the one with the small ears) carries its babies for twenty to twenty-three months. If humans had twenty-three-month pregnancies, you wouldn't even be halfway yet. For your information, the shortest pregnancies of mammals are found among opossums and an animal called the Eastern Native Cat. They carry their young for only eight to thirteen days before giving birth. Imagine having the ability to give birth two or three times a month rather than just once a year.

Full Term Plus 7

Chart your waist size and weight here.

WAIST SIZE   WEIGHT

Take care to write down the details of your baby's birth so your child can learn the story of its birthday. Do you know the story of your own birth? If you do, write it down and plan to relate it to your child when it's old enough, so your child can compare its birth to yours. If you don't know the details of your birth, ask your mother or someone else who would know.

Full Term Plus 8

Even though the baby is now one week past due, you're still well within the norm. In fact, 85% of all births are within two weeks of the estimated due date, either before or after. You and your baby just happen to be after, that's all. As long as your practitioner is satisfied with your health and the baby's there's nothing to worry about.

Full Term Plus 9

If you don't already know the sex of your baby, you might want to make your prediction now. Do you think girls or boys run in certain families? Do you have both boy and girl names picked out? What prompted you to select those names? As you amuse yourself with these exercises, remember that the baby's gender is not the most important thing about them. How your baby is doing is far more important. Continue to take steps to have a healthy baby.

If children grew up according to early indications, we should have nothing but geniuses.

J. W. GOETHE

Full Term Plus 10

If you already have children at home, spend some time planning how you will integrate this new little sister or brother into the existing family. It's important that the existing siblings don't feel threatened by the new baby. Everyone needs attention and everyone needs their own space and time to spend with family members as they choose. When the baby's old enough, teach the children how to care for, play with, lift, hug, and feed it. And then let them decide what role they will play. If they want to be a caregiver, fine. If they don't, that should be fine, too. Try to be patient and understanding with everyone's needs.

Full Term Plus 11

Where will your new baby sleep? In most of the world's cultures, babies and young children sleep in the same bed as their parents. In the United States, however, such arrangements are rare. Shared sleeping arrangements offer easy access to the child, easy breast-feeding, and more restful sleep for the baby, who enjoys the warmth and sounds of its parents. Some of the disadvantages of sharing sleep involve parents who are light sleepers, adjustments for intimacy, and the eventual weaning of the child to its own bed. Some parents worry that if the baby is in another room, they won't hear it. Unless the parent is a very deep sleeper, he or she will learn to respond to the sound of the baby's cry. You'll have to decide what arrangement best serves your needs. Sometimes the only way to know is to experiment.

A wise father doesn't see everything.
W. A. C. BENNETT

Full Term Plus 12

If you will be giving birth in a hospital or birth center, you will need a car seat to transport your baby home. Most states now have laws requiring the use of approved infant car seats. Many new mothers are tempted to hold the baby in their arms while another person operates the car, but don't—this is very dangerous. A sudden stop might wrench the baby from your arms; a sudden impact might crush the baby between you and the dashboard. Please take no risks! Purchase and use an approved car seat appropriate for a newborn and wear a seatbelt yourself at all times.

Full Term Plus 13

If you have a son, you will have to decide whether or not to have him circumcised. Circumcision is a religious rite carried out by the Muslim and Jewish faiths. Outside of religious tradition, circumcision has both advantages and disadvantages. The American Academy of Pediatrics has indicated that there is no medical advantage to routine circumcision and that good foreskin hygiene is as easy as learning to brush one's teeth. On the other hand, some people like the uniform appearance that results from circumcision even though the baby boy experiences pain during and after the procedure. About 50% of all boys in North America are circumcised. Think about it.

Full Term Plus 14

Chart your waist size and weight here.

WAIST SIZE   WEIGHT

Today marks the end of the second week past the due date. Practitioners routinely order tests of fetal well-being for babies more than two weeks overdue. The results of those tests will help direct the course of action to follow. Sometimes labor starts spontaneously after the testing, sometimes it needs a little help, sometimes it needs a lot of help. As always, remain calm and ask a lot of questions so you know what's going on. It won't be long now.

Labor and Delivery Details

When did your contractions begin to become regular?

    DATE: ....

    TIME OF DAY: ....

How far apart were these first regular contractions?

....

Had any of these events happened yet?

    CARRYING THE BABY LOW IN YOUR PELVIS? ....

    PRESSURE OR HEAVY FEELING IN THE PELVIS? ....

    BAG OF WATERS LEAKING OR BROKEN? ....

    LOSS OF THE MUCOUS PLUG? ....

    FEELING OF EXTRA ENERGY? ....

    LOSS OF WEIGHT? ....

    QUEASINESS/NAUSEA? ....

Did you call your practitioner during your labor?

    WHEN? ....

    WHAT ABOUT? ....

FOR BIRTH AT THE HOSPITAL

When did you leave to go to the hospital or birth center?

How did you get there?

How far apart were your contractions when you left?

What happened when you arrived?

What was it like?

....

....

....

....

....

....

....

....

....

....

....

....

....

FOR BIRTH AT HOME

When did your midwife arrive?

How far apart were your contractions?

What happened after the midwife arrived?

What did you do when you had contractions?

How did you manage the pain of labor?

....

....

....

....

....

....

....

....

....

....

....

....

....

....

....

When your contractions get to be two minutes apart, have someone record the sequence of events and the time at which they occurred.

CLOCK TIME: EVENT:

CLOCK TIME: EVENT:

CLOCK TIME: EVENT:

CLOCK TIME: EVENT:

REFLECTIONS ON YOUR BABY'S BIRTH

Who attended the birth of your baby?

Who played the most important role?

How did the people present react to the birth?

What kinds of things happened during labor?

What was your labor like?

How long did your labor last?

Was this labor the way you imagined it to be?

How did it compare with your expectations or with previous labors?

....

....

....

....

....

....

....

....

....

....

....

....

....

....

What kinds of things happened during the birth?

What was your experience of childbirth like?

Was childbirth the way you imagined it to be? How did it compare with your expectations or with previous births?

If you had it to do over again, what would you change about your labor and the birth of your baby?

If you had it to do over again, what aspects of labor and birth would you want to remain the same?

Who cut the baby's cord?

Did you hold the baby right after birth?

Describe your thoughts and reactions.

Did you try to nurse the baby right after birth?

Describe your experience.

IF YOU HAD A C-SECTION

Why did you have a C-section?

What did the practitioner do?

What was the hardest part of the C-section?

What was the easiest part of the C-section?

Who was there with you during the operation?

Was the C-section the way you imagined it to be?

How did your experience compare with your expectations?

....

....

....

....

....

....

....

....

....

What were the first things you noticed about your newborn baby?

What did you do, think about, or feel right after the baby was born?

....

....

....

....

Who were the first 5 people you called with the news?

....

....

How soon did you get up after giving birth?

How long did you stay in the hospital or birth center?

At home, how long did you rest before you went back to your routine?

....

....

....

....

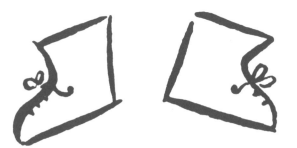

ABOUT YOUR NEW BABY

Baby's full name ....

....

How did you select the baby's name? ....

....

Date of birth ....

Time of birth ....

Weight at birth ....

Length at birth ....

What was the baby's one-minute APGAR score? ....

What was the baby's five-minute APGAR score? ....

Any hair on the baby's head? What color? ....

Any vernix (white, creamy material) on the baby's skin?

Where? ....

Any lanugo (downy hair on the body)? Where? ....

Any birthmarks? Where? ....

List any temporary changes in the baby's appearance

because of the birth (folded ear, molded head, etc.)

....

What did you like best about your baby's appearance?

What surprised you most about the baby's appearance?

....

....

....

....

....

....

....

....

Was the baby born before the due date? By how many days

or weeks? ....

Was the baby born after the due date? By how many days

or weeks? ....

What did you do the first few times you held your baby?

....

....

....

....

Breast-feeding experiences: ....

....

....

Bottle-feeding experiences: ....

....

....

Who called you "mom" for the first time? How did you

react? ....

....

What was the weather like the day the baby was born?

What local, national, or world events were in the news the
day the baby was born?

Where were you living at the time?

Who were your neighbors? Your best friends?

What type of car were you driving?

What was your favorite television show?

What were your hobbies and favorite activities?

If you were employed at the time the baby was born, what
was your job and who were you working for?

If you were a student at the time the baby was born, where
were you going to school and how far along were you
in your training?

What did you think about your whole experience of
pregnancy and childbirth?

notes

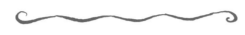

Glossary & Subject Index

A

abdomen
  baby's, 18, 28, 29, 30, 40, 48, 149, 156
  mother's, 25, 60, 67, 78, 91, 95, 127, 128, 145
abdominal pain, mother's, 63, 92, 122, 147
adrenal glands, 28; Hormone-secreting glands seated on top of the kidneys
AFP screening test, 67; Prenatal diagnostic procedure involving the detection of alphafetoprotein (AFP), a protein found in the mother's bloodstream, which diagnoses Down's syndrome and faulty development of the brain and spinal cord
air travel, 117
alcohol consumption, 12, 15, 24, 38, 71
alveoli, 20; Air sacs of the lungs
amino acid; Substance essential to the formation of protein
amniocentesis, 67; Prenatal diagnostic procedure involving the withdrawal of amniotic fluid from the womb so fetal cells can be analyzed for Down's syndrome, some metabolic and genetic disorders, and the maturity of the baby's lungs
amnion, 12, 15
amniotic cavity, 12, 13, 14; Area within the womb that contains the amniotic sac, amniotic fluid, and developing child
amniotic fluid, 12, 25, 28, 140; Fluid that surrounds and protects the developing baby
amniotic sac, 12–15, 18, 37, 106, 127, 146; Membrane that contains the amniotic fluid that cushions the developing child; also called the bag of waters or amniotic membrane
anemia, 21, 86, 87; See also iron-deficiency anemia
antibodies, 28, 53, 62, 125, 131, 155; Proteins in the blood that destroy disease-producing antigens
antioxidants, 41; Compounds that prevent other substances from breaking down, or oxidizing
anus; Exit point for solid waste; the end of the bowel, also called rectum
anvil; One of the three bones of the middle ear
aorta, 21, 31; Main artery of the heart that sends blood to all parts of the body except the lungs
APGAR; Assessment device used to evaluate the health status of the newborn baby; developed by Dr. Virginia Apgar, a pediatrician
appetite, 40, 52, 66, 141
areola, 21, 36, 37, 52, 76; Darkened, circular area that surrounds the nipple

arm buds; Tiny projections of tissue on an embryo that will later form the arms
arteries, 21, 31; Blood vessels that transport oxygen-rich blood from the lungs to the body
artificial sweeteners, 40
autonomic nervous system; Set of neurons lying along side the spinal cord that sends signals to the internal organs and glands

B

backache
  abdominal muscles and, 123
  alleviating, 63, 75–80, 82, 96
  labor and, 152
  poor posture and, 120
  severe, 124
  sleeping position and, 83
back labor, 155
bag of waters. See amniotic sac
balance, 32, 78, 121, 123, 153, 154
basal metabolism rate, 139; Base or base rate
baths
  baby, 62, 96, 98, 99, 115, 121, 125, 127, 139, 144
  maternal, 50, 121, 132
belly button, baby's, 56
bile, 51; Liquid produced by the liver and emptied into the small intestine to aid digestion
bladder, 21, 49, 63, 99, 112, 115, 149 Sac that stores the urine released from the kidneys maternal,
bladder infection, 49
bleeding
  nasal, 61
  vaginal, 12, 17
blinking, 66, 88
bloating, 19, 53, 98
blood
  circulation, 13, 58, 104, 143
  volume, 33, 38, 40, 56, 64, 135, 140
blood islands, 15, 16, 117; Groups of cells that form the baby's first red blood cells
blood pressure, 65, 104, 114, 132, 137, 144
blood sugar, 21, 87, 132
blood vessels, baby's, 13, 18, 31, 95, 98, 100, 137
bone marrow, 24, 117; Soft tissue inside the cavities and spongy portions of bones
brain, baby's, 24

Braxton-Hicks contractions, 123, 137, 145, 147, 158; "Practice" uterine contractions that do not dilate the cervix

breast feeding. See nursing

breast tenderness/changes, 17, 21, 33, 58, 95, 127

breathing
baby's, 24, 47, 52, 54, 56, 60, 92, 102, 110, 112, 113, 157
mother's, 36, 49, 86, 94, 109, 123, 127, 128, 136, 137, 150, 155

bronchi, 28; Tubes that branch from the windpipe to carry oxygen into either lung

C

caffeine, 29, 37, 38, 78, 99

caffeol, 78

calcification, 13; Process of replacing cartilage with bone; also called ossification

calcium, 13, 25, 30, 32, 37, 42, 66, 72, 74, 87, 95, 116, 121, 122

capillaries, 98; Smallest blood vessels of the body

carbohydrates, 13, 14, 26, 49, 50, 58, 69, 70; Compounds used by the body for energy, such as sugars and starches

cardiovascular system, 13; System that contains the heart and blood vessels

car seats, 135, 162

cartilage, 32, 36, 42, 81, 144; Soft tissue that hardens into bone

cell ball, 10, 11, 12

cell division, 9, 10

cephalocaudal development, 29; Development that proceeds from "head to toe" (literally, "head to tail")

cereals and grains, 14, 20, 22, 30, 33, 51, 53, 54, 55, 70, 95

cerebellum, 28; Hindbrain structure that influences complex, rapid motor movement

cerebral hemispheres, 27; Left and right halves of the brain; also called the right hemisphere and the left hemisphere

cervix, 42, 47, 79, 91, 136, 141, 143, 152; mouth of the uterus

cesarean section, 103, 130; Surgical removal of the baby from the womb; also called C-section

childbirth preparation course, 94, 157

chloride, 41; An important mineral nutrient

cholesterol, 25, 44; Fatty substance present in some foods; large amounts or poor metabolism of cholesterol can lead to artery blockage

chorion, 15

chorionic villi, 14, 16; Part of the lining of the placenta chorionic villi sampling; Prenatal diagnostic procedure in which a small piece of the chorion, or lining of the placenta, is removed for analysis to determine the baby's health and well-being in the first trimester

circulation
baby's, 13, 19, 66
mother's, 19, 48, 66, 83, 103, 104, 127, 145

circumcision, 162

clitoris, 36; Sensitive structure of the female external genitals

clumsiness, 121, 153

cm; Centimeter, a metric unit of length, equal to one-hundredth of a meter, or about 1/3 inch

colostrum, 62, 113, 125; Fluid secreted by the breasts before actual milk production begins

conception, 9, 13, 24, 92; When the chromosomes of the egg merge with those of the sperm; also called fertilization

congestion, 45, 61, 62

constipation, 53, 54, 63, 88, 126; Infrequent or difficult bowel movements

contractions, 37, 43, 87, 99, 123, 136, 137, 140, 145, 147–53, 155, 158

convolutions, 116, 125; Irregular folds on the surface of the brain

cramping
leg, 37, 79, 87, 95–96, 124, 127, 141
menstrual-like, 17, 152

cravings, 19, 61

critical period; Time during which an organ or system is growing most rapidly

D

dairy products, 13, 108

dehydration, 37, 117; Fluid loss by the body

dental health, 121, 142

diabetes, 106, 108; Metabolic disorder caused by decreased insulin production and resulting in too much sugar in the blood stream

diaphragm, 30, 109, 117, 137, 141; Muscle and connective tissue that divides the chest cavity from the abdominal cavity and is used in breathing

diarrhea, 151

diet. See nutrition

digestive system,
baby's, 12, 15, 21, 46, 47, 51, 69, 82, 100, 137

digital rays; Ridged formation on the hand plate that indicates the position of the future fingers

digits; Fingers or toes

dilation, 79, 91, 136

disease, 21–22, 34, 40, 41, 58, 131, 133, 155

dizziness. See faintness

DNA, 54; Chemical molecule (deoxyribonucleic acid) that makes up the genes

Doppler; Special listening device used to detect fetal heart sounds

G

g; Gram, a metric unit of weight and mass, roughly equal to .04 ounce

gall bladder, 21, 45, 46, 51, 147; Small sac attached to the liver that stores bile

gastrointestinal; Pertaining to the stomach and the intestines

gastrointestinal tract, 21, 131, 139

gene; Unit of heredity located on the chromosomes

genetics; Study of heredity and inherited similarities and differences

genitals, 29, 38, 52; External sex structures

germ cells, 29; Primitive forerunners of the ova or sperm

gestational diabetes; Diabetes that is only experienced during pregnancy

globulins; Natural ingredients in the blood that prevent infection

glucose, 30; blood sugar

gonads. See ovaries; testes; Sex organs; in the female, the ovaries; in the male, the testes

growth hormone; Pituitary gland secretion that stimulates bone growth

gums
baby's, 30, 50, 54, 101, 140, 142
sensitivity, 84

H

hair. See also lanugo
baby's, 15, 40, 57, 58, 79, 80, 86, 118, 124
growth, maternal, 26, 44, 78, 83

hair follicles; Small cavity or sac from which hair grows

hammer; One of the three bones of the middle ear

hand plates; Flat projections of tissue on an embryo that will form the hands

hCG (human chorionic gonadotropin), 13, 17, 48–49; Hormone secreted soon after implantation; it is detected in pregnancy tests to confirm conception

headaches, 45, 46, 114, 127, 132

hearing, baby's, 91, 97, 114, 120

heart
baby's, 13–16, 18–21, 24, 26, 30–33, 36, 37, 59, 66, 84, 85, 112
mother's, 71, 74, 77, 83, 141, 144

heartbeat
baby's, 18, 19, 24, 54, 84, 85, 97
mother's, 88

heartburn, 19, 34, 53, 98

heart tubes; Channels in an embryo that later form a primitive heart

hemorrhoids, 88, 100, 101; Enlarged veins in the lower part of the rectum

herbicides, 63

hindbrain, 24; The most posterior part of the brain including the pons, medulla, and cerebellum

hormone; Any of several substances secreted into the blood stream by endocrine glands. They affect the activity of organs

hormone levels, 13, 20, 29, 31, 48–49, 53, 61, 62, 66, 84, 98, 159

hygiene, 29, 96, 99, 108, 111, 121

I

immune system, 9, 54, 131, 133, 155, 157

implantation, 10–13, 17; When the fertilized egg burrows into the lining of the uterus, where it will be nourished and protected until birth

indigestion, 19, 34, 53, 72, 98, 117

infection, 34, 49, 62, 70, 81, 99, 108, 112, 131

inner ear; Portion of the ear that detects motion (semicircular canals) and sends information about sound to the brain via the auditory nerve

insulin, 51, 54, 107; Hormone secreted by the pancreas that regulates the body's use of sugar and other carbohydrates

intercourse, 93, 115, 143

intestines, 21, 25, 29, 34, 38, 48, 50, 51, 97, 147; Part of the digestive system that absorbs nutrients and water and excretes waste

inversion, 130; Technique designed to reposition the fetus in utero so it will be head-down at birth

iodine, 53, 96; Essential mineral nutrient

iris, 42, 123; Colored portion of the eye

iron; Essential mineral nutrient
absorption of, 41
importance of, 33, 69, 87, 116, 121, 138
sources of, 20, 46, 47, 48, 50, 62, 70, 86

iron deficiency anemia, 86, 87; Condition caused by an iron-poor diet in which fewer red blood cells develop and those that are present carry less oxygen to the cells

IU International unit; a unit of measurement

J

jaws, baby's, 19, 27, 30

K

Kegel exercises, 28

kg; Kilogram, a metric unit of weight and mass, equal to 1,000 grams (and roughly equal to two pounds)

kidneys, 22, 24, 26, 31, 36, 44, 48, 58, 74, 100, 112; Organ that filters certain wastes out of the blood stream and forms urine